Tumor Virus Infections
and Immunity

Proceedings of a Symposium on Tumor Virus Infections and Immunity, held under the auspices of the Eastern Pennsylvania Branch of the American Society for Microbiology, in Philadelphia, April 24-25, 1975

Program Chairmen:

Richard L. Crowell, Ph.D.
Herman Friedman, Ph.D.

Symposium Sponsors:

Eastern Pennsylvania Branch,
American Society for
  Microbiology,
Philadelphia, PA

Bureau of Laboratories,
Pennsylvania Department of
  Health,
Philadelphia, PA

Department of Microbiology,
Temple University Medical
  School,
Philadelphia, PA

Department of Microbiology,
Hahnemann Medical College
  and Hospital,
Philadelphia, PA

Contributors:

Burroughs Welcome Company
Research Triangle Park, NC

Damon Corporation
Needham Heights, MA

Endo Laboratories of E.I. Dupont
  de Nemours Company
Garden City, NY

Flow Laboratories
Rockville, MD

Grand Island Biological Co.
  (GIBCO)
Chagrin Falls, OH

ICI United States, Inc.
Wilmington, DE

Lederle Laboratories Division,
  American Cyanamid Co.
Pearl River, NY

Merck, Sharpe, and Dohme Co.
West Point, PA

Microbiological Associates
Bethesda, MD

Ortho Pharmaceutical Corp.
Raritan, NJ

Smith Kline Diagnostics
Philadelphia, PA

Previously published volumes in the series of symposia sponsored by the Eastern Pennsylvania Branch of the American Society for Microbiology:

AUSTRALIA ANTIGEN (Proceedings of the Third Annual Symposium, edited by James E. Prier and Herman Friedman)

OPPORTUNISTIC PATHOGENS (Proceedings of the Fourth Annual Symposium, edited by James E. Prier and Herman Friedman)

QUALITY CONTROL IN MICROBIOLOGY (Proceedings of the Fifth Annual Symposium, edited by James E. Prier, Josephine T. Bartola, and Herman Friedman)

MODERN METHODS IN MEDICAL MICROBIOLOGY (Proceedings of the Sixth Annual Symposium, edited by James E. Prier, Josephine T. Bartola, and Herman Friedman)

Tumor Virus Infections and Immunity

Edited by

Richard L. Crowell, Ph.D.
Hahnemann Medical College

Herman Friedman, Ph.D.
Albert Einstein Medical Center, Temple University

James E. Prier, D.V.M., Ph.D.
Pennsylvania Bureau of Laboratories

University Park Press
Baltimore • London • Tokyo

UNIVERSITY PARK PRESS
International Publishers in Science and Medicine
Chamber of Commerce Building
Baltimore, Maryland 21202

Copyright © 1976 by University Park Press
Typeset by Service Composition, Baltimore, Maryland
Manufactured in the United States of America
by Universal Lithographers, Inc., and The Maple Press Co.

616.994

S y 68 T

Library of Congress Cataloging in Publication Data
ASM Symposium on Tumor Virus Infections and Immunity,
Philadelphia, 1975.
Tumor virus infections and immunity.

Includes index.
1. Viral carcinogenesis—Congresses. 2. Tumors—
Immunological aspects—Congresses. 3. Oncogenic viruses
—Congresses.   I. Crowell, Richard Lane.   II. Friedman,
Herman, 1931-   III. Prier, James E.   IV. American
Society for Microbiology. Eastern Pennsylvania Branch.

V. Title.
RC268.57.A18 1975   616.9'94'0194   76-10688
ISBN 0-8391-0891-5

Contents

120192

Participants

J. T. August, M.D.
Department of Molecular Biology
Albert Einstein College of Medicine
   of Yeshiva University
Bronx, New York

Laure Aurelian, Ph.D.
Departments of Laboratory
   Animal Medicine, Biochemistry
   and Biophysics, and Microbiology
The Johns Hopkins University
   School of Medicine
Baltimore, Maryland

Robert B. Bell, Ph.D.
Department of Laboratory
   Animal Medicine
The Johns Hopkins University
   School of Medicine
Baltimore, Maryland

Mauro Bendinelli, Ph.D.
Department of Microbiology
Albert Einstein Medical Center,
   Temple University
Philadelphia, Pennsylvania

John A. Bilello, Ph.D.
Department of Molecular Biology
Albert Einstein College of Medicine
   of Yeshiva University
Bronx, New York

Guy D. Bonnard, M.D.
Laboratory of Immunodiagnosis
National Cancer Institute
National Institutes of Health
Bethesda, Maryland

Walter S. Ceglowski, Ph.D.
Department of Microbiology
   and Cell Biology
The Pennsylvania State University
   College of Medicine
University Park, Pennsylvania

S. Chandra, M.D.
Mercy Hospital
Chicago, Illinois

Carlo M. Croce, M.D.
The Wistar Institute of Anatomy
   and Biology
Philadelphia, Pennsylvania

Jeffrey G. Derge, Ph.D.
Flow Laboratories
Rockville, Maryland

Paul A. Farber, Ph.D.
Department of Pathology
Temple University School
   of Dentistry
Philadelphia, Pennsylvania

Herman Friedman, Ph.D.
Department of Microbiology
Albert Einstein Medical Center,
   Temple University
Philadelphia, Pennsylvania

Philip Furmanski, Ph.D.
Cell Biology Laboratory
Michigan Cancer Foundation
Detroit, Michigan

Dario Giacomoni, Ph.D.
Department of Microbiology
University of Illinois at the
   Medical Center
Chicago, Illinois

Moshe Glaser, Ph.D.
Laboratory of Immunodiagnosis
National Cancer Institute
National Institutes of Health
Bethesda, Maryland

Berge Hampar, D.D.S.
Laboratory of DNA Tumor Viruses
National Cancer Institute
National Institutes of Health
Bethesda, Maryland

M. G. Hanna, Jr., Ph.D.
Basic Research Program
Frederick Cancer Research Center
Frederick, Maryland

Stephen Haskill, Ph.D.
Departments of Basic and Clinical
   Immunology and Microbiology
Medical University of
   South Carolina
Charleston, South Carolina

P. Heller, M.D.
Veterans Administration Hospital
   West Side, and Departments of
   Microbiology and Medicine
University of Illinois at the
   Medical Center
Chicago, Illinois

Ronald B. Herberman, M.D.
Laboratory of Immunodiagnosis
National Cancer Institute
National Institutes of Health
Bethesda, Maryland

Martin S. Hirsch, M.D.
Massachusetts General Hospital
Harvard Medical School
Boston, Massachusetts

Howard T. Holden, Ph.D.
Laboratory of Immunodiagnosis
National Cancer Institute
National Institutes of Health
Bethesda, Maryland

Cheng-Po Hu, Ph.D.
Department of Microbiology
   and Immunology
Temple University School
   of Medicine
Philadelphia, Pennsylvania

James N. Ihle, Ph.D.
Basic Research Program
Frederick Cancer Research Center
Frederick, Maryland

Robert P. Jacobs, M.D.
Departments of Medicine
   and Epidemiology
The Johns Hopkins University
   School of Medicine
   and School of Hygiene
   and Public Health
Baltimore, Maryland

J. Katzmann, Ph.D.
Department of Microbiology
University of Illinois at the
   Medical Center
Chicago, Illinois

Holger Kirchner, M.D.
Laboratory of Immunodiagnosis
National Cancer Institute
National Institutes of Health
Bethesda, Maryland

Gundula U. LaBadie, M.S.
Department of Microbiology
   and Cell Biology
The Pennsylvania State University
   College of Medicine
University Park, Pennsylvania

Kenneth M. Lam, Ph.D.
Department of Microbiology
 and Immunology
Temple University School
 of Medicine
Philadelphia, Pennsylvania

John C. Lee, Ph.D.
Basic Research Program
Frederick Cancer Research Center
Frederick, Maryland

T. Juhani Linna, M.D., Ph.D.
Department of Microbiology
 and Immunology
Temple University School
 of Medicine
Philadelphia, Pennsylvania

Janice D. Longstreth, M.S.
Basic Research Program
Frederick Cancer Research Center
Frederick, Maryland

Afework A. Mascio, Ph.D.
Department of Microbiology
 and Cell Biology
The Pennsylvania State University
University Park, Pennsylvania

Justin J. McCormick, Ph.D.
Molecular Biology Laboratory
Michigan Cancer Foundation
Detroit, Michigan

Charles M. McGrath, Ph.D.
Tumor Biology Laboratory
Michigan Cancer Foundation
Detroit, Michigan

Dan H. Moore, Ph.D., D.Sc. (Hon.)
Institute for Medical Research
Camden, New Jersey

Navin Patel, Ph.D.
Department of Microbiology
Albert Einstein Medical Center,
 Temple University
Philadelphia, Pennsylvania

Herbert J. Rapp, Sc.D.
Biology Branch
National Cancer Institute
National Institutes of Health
Bethesda, Maryland

Marvin A. Rich, Ph.D.
Michigan Cancer Foundation and
 Wayne State University School
 of Medicine
Detroit, Michigan

Jose Russo, M.D.
Experimental Pathology Laboratory
Michigan Cancer Foundation
Detroit, Michigan

Stuart Z. Shapiro, Ph.D.
Department of Molecular Biology
Albert Einstein College of Medicine
 of Yeshiva University
Bronx, New York

Marie F. Smith, B.A.
Department of Laboratory
 Animal Medicine
The Johns Hopkins University
 School of Medicine
Baltimore, Maryland

Steven Specter, Ph.D.
Department of Microbiology
Albert Einstein Medical Center,
 Temple University
Philadelphia, Pennsylvania

Bruce C. Strand, Ph.D.
Department of Laboratory
 Animal Medicine
The Johns Hopkins University
 School of Medicine
Baltimore, Maryland

Mette Strand, Ph.D.
Department of Molecular Biology
Albert Einstein College of Medicine
 of Yeshiva University
Bronx, New York

Kenneth D. Thompson, Ph.D.
Department of Microbiology
and Immunology
Temple University School
of Medicine
Philadelphia, Pennsylvania

George J. Todaro, M.D.
Viral Oncology Program
National Cancer Institute
National Institutes of Health
Bethesda, Maryland

Preface

Malignant neoplastic disease represents the culmination of a sequence of events initiated by viruses or other agents and moderated by the immune response of the host. Experimentation in cancer research over the past several decades has led to the development of numerous hypotheses in an attempt to account for the etiology and expression of malignancies. While the putative role of viruses as causative agents of human neoplastic disease has not been proven as yet, there exists a voluminous body of literature concerning the interrelationships between viruses, the immune system, and malignancy in sub-human primates and lower animals. Thus, the organizers of this symposium considered it timely to bring together prominent investigators from the fields of tumor virology and tumor immunology, whose presentation of their recent research findings would help to provide direction and insight into this complex problem.

The dual processes of neoplastic transformation of cells by viruses and the effect of the immunologic state of the host before, during, and following transformation constitute the focus of this publication. It is apparent that the immunologic response of the host to neoplasia is multifaceted and contributes to resolution of the disease or, alternatively, to the ultimate demise of the host.

It is appropriate that tumor virus infections be viewed, at least in part, as models of infectious diseases with which there are many parallels in a classic sense. For example, viruses or their nucleic acids are transmissible agents, and the outcome of their infections depends on the capacity of the immune response to control them. In addition, attention must be given to the many newly acquired properties of transformed cells that distinguish them from normal cells. It is hoped that the contributions reported herein will bring together the thoughts of the virologists and the immunologists whose cooperative efforts are needed to deal more effectively with human neoplasms.

This symposium, held under the auspices of the Eastern Pennsylvania Branch of the American Society for Microbiology, provided a forum for the exchange of information among the participants and the more than 200 persons who attended. The topics discussed included the nature and biological activities of DNA and RNA tumor viruses, the effects of these viruses on a variety of host species, and the nature of the immune responses to these viruses and the tumors they induce. More specifically, the reports included in this symposium dealt with: the emerging recognition of the role of members of the herpesvirus group as possible human cancer agents; the recognition of tumor virus genes being located on specific chromosomes and that they may have resided in the hereditary gene pool of primates down through the centuries; the finding of type C oncornavirus-induced gene expressions as antigens of normal and diseased human tissues; the recognition of autogenous immunity to endogenous tumor viruses; and with viruses and breast cancer of mice and humans, a progress report on the development of a virus vaccine. In subsequent sessions, numerous informative reports were given on the phenomena of suppression of both humoral and cell-mediated immune responses by leukemia viruses, and of the immune activation of endogenous tumor viruses. Of potential therapeutic significance, the effects of non-specific enhancement and/or stimulation of immune responsiveness to leukemia viruses as mediated by BCG were also discussed. The information was presented in a manner which could be readily understood by the audience, who were mostly microbiologists involved in a variety of academic and clinical laboratory endeavors. The discussion after each of the papers was wide ranging, and it indicated to all that further advances in the exciting area of tumor virus infection and immunity soon will be forthcoming.

ACKNOWLEDGMENTS

On behalf of all participating in this conference we extend our gratitude and appreciation to the many individuals and sponsoring organizations who made this symposium possible. Additionally, we are grateful to Barbara Zajac, Vittorio Defendi, Wallace Rowe, George Todaro, Juhanni Linna, and Chester Southam, who served as session moderators and/or discussers.

Richard L. Crowell
Herman Friedman
James E. Prier
Philadelphia
March, 1976

Tumor Virus Infections and Immunity

CHAPTER 1

Genetic Expression of Mammalian RNA Tumor Viruses

M. Strand, J. A. Bilello,
S. Z. Shapiro, and J. T. August

I. INTRODUCTION

RNA type C tumor viruses show two remarkable properties. One is that at least one gene product of these viruses is involved in malignant transformation of the infected cell. This property has stimulated widespread interest in these viruses for studies of the mechanism of carcinogenesis, because it provides a means to apply genetic, as well as biological and biochemical techniques to the analysis of onco-genesis. Second, it is known that the genome of type C RNA tumor viruses is present as an endogenous genetic component of the cells of many, if not all, animals and is transmitted from parent to progeny along with other cellular genes (24, 25, 27, 30, 50, 56, 67). These viral genes appear to be a hereditary component of an animal's normal genetic endowment and it may be that the virus evolved from the cell (67). As such, the expression of this gene information is obviously under the control of the host cell and may well occur as a normal function of the cell. These viruses thus offer unique experimental opportunities for studies of genetic expression in eukaryotic cells. They provide a relatively simple means to obtain the RNA transcripts of cellular genes and many of the structural products of these genes, and they make possible specific genetic analysis of these genes.

1

II. VIRAL GENE PRODUCTS

Currently, the bulk of the evidence suggests that the viral genome contains one or identical 35 S subunits of about 3×10^6 daltons (6, 12, 15, 33, 74). If this is correct, there could be about 300,000 daltons of viral coded protein.

Most viral gene products appear to be structural proteins of the virion. Purified virions of mammalian RNA type C viruses may contain as many as 50 polypeptides (Figure 1). Because the sum of the apparent molecular weights of these polypeptides is much

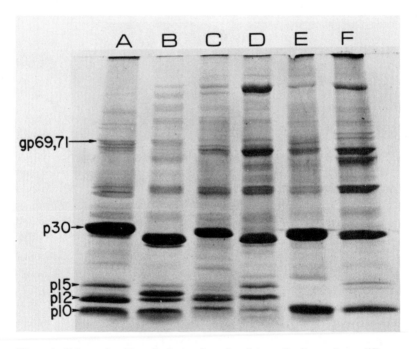

Figure 1. Polyacrylamide gel electrophoresis of type C viruses from different mammalian species in a high resolution, 7.5–20% gradient polyacrylamide slab gel in the presence of 0.1% SDS. (A) Kirsten murine sarcoma virus, 66 μg, propagated in normal rat kidney cells. (B) Rat leukemia virus, 68 μg, propagated in Lewis rat embryo fibroblasts (Kelment et al. 1973). (C) Hamster leukemia virus, 72 μg, propagated in hamster embryo fibroblasts (Kelloff et al. 1970. (D) Theilen feline leukemia virus, 70 μg, propagated in the FL74 cat lymphoblastoid cells (Theilen et al. 1969). (E) RD-114 virus, 68 μg, propagated in human rhabdomyosarcoma (RD cells) (McAllister et al. 1972). (F) SSV-1 (woolly monkey virus), 70 μg, propagated in NC-37 human lymphocyte cells.

greater than that which could be coded by the viral genome, it is apparent that many derive from the host cell or tissue culture medium. Several have been identified as virus-specific, chiefly from the finding that their concentration is greatly increased following virus infection, and also by immunochemical analysis. The chief component is a protein of approximately 27,000–30,000 molecular weight (p27–p30), the major structural protein of the virus. This polypeptide comprises 10–20% of the total protein of the virion and is found in all mammalian type C viruses. Another major component is the viral envelope glycopeptides of apparent molecular weight about 70,000 (gp70). This glycopeptide is not readily distinguished by polyacrylamide gel analysis because of the presence of other (contaminating) proteins of similar molecular weight, and in some cases of bovine serum albumin. However, by immunochemical analysis, an analogous component with cross-reactive antigenic determinants has been found in all other viruses tested, including the feline, RD 114, and woolly monkey groups (58, 59). Another known, but minor, viral component of about 70,000 daltons is the reverse transcriptase (1, 21, 37, 73), which has been shown by genetic experiments to be viral coded (35). Several low molecular weight proteins are also present in the virions, and for the murine viruses they have been characterized as components of about 15,000 (p15), 12,000 (p12), and 10,000 (p10) daltons. Proteins of 15,000 (63) and 12,000 daltons (69) have been purified and found to be virus-specific by the presence of type-specific determinants as the main antigenic component. Analogous components in viruses of different groups are not distinguished by their size (Figure 1), and even in different types of murine viruses marked variation in the small molecular weight protein is observed (59). In the case of the p15 component, however, the presence of analogous proteins in different viruses was shown by group and interspecies antigenic cross-reactivity (63). Ultimately, the identity of these low molecular weight proteins in different viruses will depend upon their isolation and immunochemical characterization, because size alone is not sufficiently characteristic. It can be expected that the results will be complex. For example, Parks et al. (48) reported that 12,000- and 10,000-dalton proteins of Moloney murine leukemia virus are closely related and we (Strand and August, unpublished) have found a 12,000-dalton protein of

(9, 17, 41). A drawback of this procedure, however, is protein denaturation, which may modify the chemical and biological properties of the proteins (29). An additional problem is that relatively little attention has been given to the recovery of protein and, in general, the yield of purified components appears to have been low.

Several of the viral polypeptides are known to express interspecies antigenic determinants cross-reactive with analogous proteins of type C viruses of other species (19, 20). Of the major structural proteins of the virion, three have been found to demonstrate such reactivity, the core protein of 30,000 daltons (22), the envelope glycoprotein (58), and the internal protein of 15,000 daltons (63). In the purification of virion proteins particular attention has been given to these three because of the demonstrated utility of the interspecies determinants to make possible the use of a protein of one type of species of virus to measure that of another. Moreover, in the initial phases of this work the interspecies reactivity of these proteins provides a means for relatively selective assay procedures.

An important consideration has been to achieve a high yield of purified protein. Moreover, to make use of these proteins for studies of the biologic and immunologic properties of the virus, conditions for purification were selected to preserve the native conformation of the proteins. These criteria have been achieved using column chromatographic procedures with approximately 50% overall yield of each of the three proteins from the same batch of virus (62). The purified fractions are highly homogeneous, as shown by polyacrylamide gel electrophoresis (Figure 2).

As a further test of protein purity and antigenic specificity, each protein was tested for contamination by the others, using antisera prepared against each of the purified components. The individual monospecific antiserum precipitated only the homologous protein at titers of 10^3–10^4 and there was no precipitation of the others, even with undiluted serum (Table 1).

Evidence for the successful recovery of active proteins by this procedure has come from the many studies using antisera prepared against the purified proteins (8, 29, 55, 58, 59, 63, 64, 71, 72, 76).

B.   Characterization of the Viral Envelope Glycopeptides

   1. Chemical Properties   The purified gp69/71 fraction contains carbohydrate residues, indicating that the polypeptides comprise

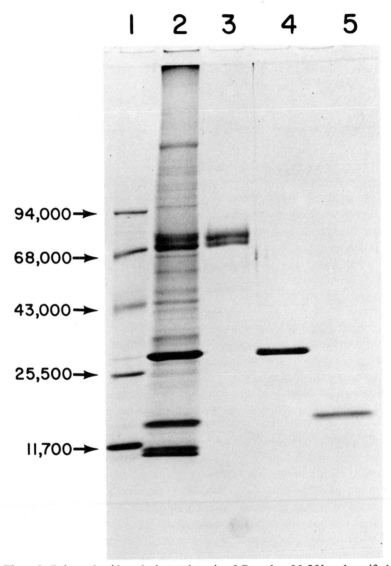

Figure 2. Polyacrylamide gel electrophoresis of Rauscher MuLV and purified viral proteins. (*1*) Standard proteins: cytochrome *c* (3.3 μg, MW 11,700); chymotrypsinogen (3.3 μg, MW 25,500); ovalbumin (4.2 μg, MW 43,000); bovine serum albumin (2.5 μg, MW 68,000); phosphorylase A (6.6 μg, MW 94,000); (*2*) Rauscher MuLV, 80 μg of protein; (*3*) purified Rauscher MuLV gp69/71, 9.4 μg of protein; (*4*) purified Rauscher MuLV p30, 3.4 μg of protein; (*5*) purified Rauscher MuLV p15, 10.5 μg of protein.

Table 1. Antigenic specificity of Rauscher murine virus p15, p30, and gp69/71[a]

	Antiserum[c] (titer)		
Antigen[b]	anti-p15	anti-p30	anti-gp69/71
^{125}I-p15	3,000	12	12
^{125}I-p30	12	36,000	12
^{125}I-gp69/71	12	12	60,000

[a]The specificity and purity of the proteins and antiserum prepared against each was tested by radioimmunoassay.

[b]Proteins were purified and radiolabeled as described in the text.

[c]Goat antiserum obtained by immunizing with the purified fractions was prepared as described in "Methods." The assays were carried out with 4 ng ^{125}I-p15 (4.4 $\times$ 10^4 cpm/ng), 1 ng ^{125}I-p30 (4.0 $\times$ 10^4 cpm/ng), and 2 ng ^{125}I-gp69/71 (4.8 $\times$ 10^4 cpm/ng).

glycoprotein components of the virus. Analysis of both disrupted virions and the purified gp69/71 by polyacrylamide gel electrophoresis, followed by staining with the Schiff-periodate reagent, shows that these components, constituting 5–10% of the total protein of purified virions, are the major glycoprotein constituents of the virion. Both the 69,000- and 71,000-dalton moieties contain sugars.

It has not yet been determined whether the two closely related glycopeptides comprising this component contain two different proteins, or the same protein with differences in the amount or composition of the sugar residues. Results favoring the interpretation that the proteins are identical are that the two cannot be distinguished by antisera prepared with other murine viruses, or viruses of other species; this indicates that they contain identical or highly similar group and interspecies antigenic determinants. This point is extremely important, for if the two glycoproteins represented different polypeptides, it would provide strong implications that a more complex genome exists or that the preparation originated from two different viruses.

Because the migration of glycoproteins in sodium dodecyl sulfate-polyacrylamide gel electrophoresis may not be an accurate measurement of size, the molecular weights of 69,000 and 71,000 of the two glycopeptides may be in excess of the true values. Other estimates of molecular weight are 70,000, obtained by gel filtration in guanidine-HCl (*40*), and 58,000, obtained by sedimentation analysis (*38*).

A frequent question has been whether the antigenic determinants reside in the protein or carbohydrate fraction of the molecules. The evidence suggests that the character of the determinants is specified by the protein. This is because the antigenic specificities of gp69/71 remain the same when the virus is propagated in cells of widely differing species and are thus virus-specific. For the determinants to be specified by the carbohydrate moiety, additional viral gene products would be required for synthesis of the type- and group-specific determinants of the molecules.

2. *Viral Envelope Localization*   The envelope localization of gp69/71 in the virion has been demonstrated by use of several selective techniques to label virion surface components. Terminal sialic acid of glycoproteins was labeled by borohydride reduction after specific enzymatic or chemical oxidation and the exposed tyrosine residues of surface proteins were labeled by enzymatic iodination. In every case, the major component labeled was the gp69/71, as confirmed by immunoprecipitation with monospecific antiserum. Thus it appears that the outer envelope of the type C virus may be wholly or chiefly comprised of a single component. It may also be concluded that gp69/71 was the envelope glycoprotein labeled by lactoperoxidase iodination and demonstrated on surfaces of intact virions and infected cells (*32, 75*). It also corresponds to the major glycoprotein precipitated by sera of mice reacting against their endogenous type C viruses (*28*).

The finding that the gp69/71 is the major viral envelope component is of exceptional interest because of the possible expression of this viral gene component as a cell surface constituent in virus-producing or transformed cells. Such expression does, in fact, occur as the G_{ix} cell surface constituent and with certain sarcoma virus-infected cells (see below).

3. *Virus Neutralization*   Both rabbit and goat monospecific antisera to gp69/71 showed strong virus neutralizing activity, in keeping with the occurrence of gp69/71 as the major envelope glycoprotein. This was demonstrated both with the spleen focus-forming assay and with the XC-plaque assay (*55*). Neutralization was demonstrated not only with Rauscher virus, but also with several other murine viruses tested, including endogenous ecotropic and xenotropic viruses, suggesting that group as well as type

determinants of gp69/71 are recognized in neutralization. An alternative interpretation is that the Rauscher virus propagated in JLS-V9 cells is contaminated with an endogenous BALB/c virus and that the purified gp69/71 contains both Rauscher and BALB/c virus envelope components.

This purification and identification of the major viral neutralization determinants has considerable relevance to studies of the possible treatment of viral infection by vaccination. If such treatment were possible, consideration should be given to using a subviral component as the vaccine. Based on our findings, this subviral product would be the gp69/71 or some antigenically active derivative.

4. Antigenic Properties Each of the three classes of antigenic determinants, type, group, and interspecies, is exhibited by gp69/71 when measured by the competition radioimmunoassay (*59*). In the case of the interspecies determinants measured in a murine gp69/71: anti-feline virus serum system, equal inhibition was observed with every murine virus tested, indicating that the concentrations and affinities of the interspecies determinants of the gp69/71 proteins of these different types of murine viruses were the same. This finding is particularly important, because it provides a procedure whereby the purified protein of Rauscher virus can be used as a quantitative assay of the analogous protein of other murine viruses. Such a quantitative assay could not be carried out with a homologous assay system, because the type-specific differences of the murine virus gp69/71 protein result in as much as a 10-fold difference in the concentrations or affinities of the group determinants of the protein from different viruses. Much of our work with this protein as a probe for viral gene expression is based upon this heterologous assay.

Extensive characterization has shown that these interspecies determinants are a property of the gp69/71 and not some contaminating protein (*58*). Additionally, it is apparent that these antigenic determinants of the gp69/71 are completely distinct from those of other proteins, because there are no cross-reactive determinants between the three viral polypeptides.

5. Evidence that the gp69/71 is Virus Coded An explicit demonstration that a given protein is virus-specific can be provided by genetic or translational experiments. These experiments are yet not possible, however, and in the absence of such evidence another approach is to determine whether the antigenic determinants of the protein are viral-specific or host-specific. For this purpose we have compared the type- and group-specific determinants of gp69/71 of Rauscher MuLV propagated in JLS-V9 mouse cells, normal rat kidney cells, human embryonic kidney, and a human lymphoblast-derived line (NC-37). In the competition radioimmunoassay with ^{125}I-gp69/71 as antigen and the homologous monospecific antiserum, viruses grown in the different cells were equally efficient in competing for antibody binding in respect to all three parameters of the radio-immunoassay: the concentration of antigens, the affinity of antibody binding, and the composition of determinants. Because the assay measures virus type and group-specific determinants of the proteins, it provides strong, if not conclusive, evidence of viral coding of gp69/71. In keeping with this finding, the concentration of gp69/71 is greatly (100- to 1,000-fold) increased in cells producing virus.

6. Cell Surface Expression   The finding that the gp69/71 is the major viral envelope component led directly to the consideration of the possible expression of this viral gene component as a cell surface constituent in virus-producing or transformed cells. This has now been demonstrated in a variety of ways:

Immunofluorescence Analysis   The initial evidence that the gp69/71 components are expressed on the surface of cells came from immunofluorescence studies (*29*). Using membrane immuno-fluorescence and immunofluorescence absorption procedures with both intact and disrupted cells, these studies demonstrated the anti-genic determinants of gp69/71 on the cell surface as well as in the cytoplasm of productively infected cells.

External Labeling of Cells   An analysis of murine virus-related proteins associated with the cell surface was done. External iodina-tion by lactoperoxidase of normal and malignant thymocytes from mice, followed by immuneprecipitation and analysis of immune complexes by sodium dodecyl sulfate gel electrophoresis, showed the presence of a glycoprotein of 70,000 daltons analogous to gp69/71 (*13*).

Analysis of Cells Infected with a Defective Virus   It could be argued that the presence of the glycoprotein on the cell surface of "normal" cells was due to the budding of viruses, perhaps noninfec-tious or at very low titer. A direct demonstration that the viral envelope protein can be present on the cell surface in the absence of budding viruses has come from examination of cells infected by defective viruses.

Recently we have identified a class of defective sarcoma virus expressing gp69/71 (8). In studies using normal rat kidney cells infected by a nonmutagenized stock of Kirsten sarcoma and leukemia virus complex, two classes of nonproductive, transformed cells were found: One class synthesized the major envelope glycoprotein gp69/71 at a concentration equal to that of productively transformed cells, but showed no detectable synthesis of the major structural proteins p30 and p15; the other class did not direct the synthesis of any of the three polypeptides. External labeling of the protein or sugar moieties of the gp69/71 positive cells followed by immunoprecipitation with anti-gp69/71 serum indicated that the viral glycoprotein was present on the cell surface. Perhaps even stronger evidence of this has come from analysis of the interference properties of the cells. The sarcoma genome of cells expressing gp69/71 was not rescuable by superinfection with other murine leukemia viruses. In contrast, the sarcoma genome of both gp69/71 expressor and gp69/71 nonexpressor cells could efficiently be rescued by superinfection with a woolly monkey virus. This restriction to rescue by murine leukemia virus appeared to be localized to cell surface interactions, as the block to murine leukemia rescue could be overcome by Sendai virus mediated cell fusion of the gp69/71 expressor cells to a murine leukemia virus-producing cell line. These interference properties thus provide strong evidence for cell surface expression of gp69/71 in cells where there is no evidence of virus expression even when analyzed by sensitive immunochemical techniques.

Characterization of the G_{ix} Cell Surface Antigen as a Property of gp69/71   One of the known cell surface antigenic determinants is G_{ix}. This antigen is expressed on the thymocytes of some strains of mice (57). In the absence of virus synthesis, G_{ix} depends on the T-lymphocyte pathway of differentiation and is not found with other cells, with the exception of sperm (10, 42, 43). Cells producing murine viruses may express G_{ix} on their surface regardless of their tissue type or their inherited G_{ix} genotype, suggesting that the G_{ix^+} character of mouse thymocytes represents partial expression of the murine virus genome (42). In 129 mice its expression was shown to be dependent on two loci of chromosomes 7 and 17 (56, 57). One of these genes is *GV-1*, which appears to be distantly linked to H-2 in chromosome 17. Stockert et al. have developed two congenic mouse strains from the $129_{G_{ix}^+} \times$ C57BL/$6_{G_{ix}^-}$ cross: (1) $129_{G_{ix}^-}$, which carries the negative allele of GV-1 from B6 on a 129 background and (2) $B6_{G_{ix}^+}$, which carries the positive allele of GV-1 from 129 on a B6 background (56).

Recently, in collaboration with Lilly, we found that spleen cells of strains 129, B6 and $B6_{G_{ix}^+}$ demonstrated low to moderate levels of gp69/71 and p30, but that cells from $129_{G_{ix}^-}$ mice showed no detectable levels of either protein (65, 66). Furthermore, tissues of F_1 crosses of $129_{G_{ix}^-}$ with AKR and with DBA/2 contained significant levels of both proteins, indicating that their absence in $129_{G_{ix}^-}$ mice is a recessive trait. Since the congenic 129 and $129_{G_{ix}^-}$ strains presumably differ only with respect to a short chromosomal segment that includes the *GV-1* locus, it appears that this chromosomal segment includes the determinants not only of G_{ix}, but also of the gp69/71 and p30. The apparent close linkage of these three classes of murine antigenic determinants (G_{ix}, gp69/71, and p30) in the *GV-1* region strongly suggests that a chromosomally integrated "V" gene, perhaps incomplete since these mice do not express infectious viruses, is the basis for these observations; strain 129 mice possess this "V" gene, whereas $129_{G_{ix}^-}$ mice do not. However, it remained to explain why B6 mice, which lack the *GV-1* associated "V" gene, are nevertheless positive when tested for gp69/71 and p30. It was hypothesized that G_{ix} is a type-specific determinant of the gp69/71 protein coded for by a gene of strain 129 and other G_{ix}^+ mice, termed the *GV-1* gene, but not a determinant of gp69/71 or B6 or other G_{ix}^- mice coded for by a different "V" gene (*GV-X*). $B6_{G_{ix}^+}$ mice would thus possess both *GV-1* and *GV-X,* which is in accordance with the observation that these mice show a higher level of gp69/71 than either B6 or 129 mice, which possess *GV-1* or *GV-X,* but not both (66).

This hypothesis was strongly supported by the findings of Obata et al., who demonstrated that G_{ix} and gp69/71 were physically inseparable (42). They also showed that if the thymocytes of a mouse strain expressed G_{ix} on their surfaces, then both G_{ix} and gp69/71 antigens were present in their serum. Although other soluble murine virus antigens, FMR and GSA, have previously been demonstrated free in serum, this has only been so in mice producing large quantities of virus, whereas the presence of G_{ix} antigen in serum is independent of virus output. A critical experiment was the absorption of the G_{ix} antigen from the serum of mice by immunoprecipitation with the goat anti-Rauscher gp69/71 serum. After removal of the immunocomplexes the supernatant was tested for residual G_{ix} activity by the cytotoxic assay and for gp69/71 activity by the indirect immunofluorescence absorption assay. The result of such an absorption was that the G_{ix} as well as the gp69/71 antigenic determinants were removed, thus providing strong evidence that they both are expressed by the same molecule. The goat anti-Rauscher gp69/71 serum was also tested and found to demonstrate a weak, but nevertheless specific, cytotoxicity in the 129 thymocyte cytotoxic assay. One possibility for the weakness of this reaction could be that the reaction is strictly on a group-specific basis (anti-Rauscher gp69/71 serum and strain 129 thymocytes) and, as shown by the antigenic characterization of gp69/71, the group-specific reactivity accounts for less than 50% of the total reactivity of the serum.

Other evidence of the linkage of the G_{ix} thymocyte surface antigen to the gp69/71 envelope glycoprotein of murine virus was obtained by Tung et al. (71). Cells from $129_{G_{ix}^+}$ and $129_{G_{ix}^-}$ strains of mice were labeled with ^{125}iodine or [^{3}H]glucosamine. The labeled proteins were immunoprecipitated with cytotoxic G_{ix} serum or the goat anti-Rauscher gp69/71 serum and analyzed by sodium dodecyl sulfate polyacrylamide gel electrophoresis. It was found that regardless of the antiserum used, a protein of 70,000 daltons was present on the thymocytes of the $129_{G_{ix}^+}$ strain of mice, but never on the thymocytes from the $129_{G_{ix}^-}$ strain of mice. This 70,000-dalton protein comigrated with the envelope protein immunoprecipitated from ^{125}I-labeled or [^{3}H]glucosamine-labeled intact virus.

Additional evidence has been presented that G_{ix} is a type-specific determinant of gp69/71 (72). By use of assay procedures identical to those in their earlier work described above, thymocytes of 129, $B6_{G_{ix}^-}$, and $B6_{G_{ix}^+}$ were compared for the coexpression of G_{ix} and gp69/71. B6, although it is gp69/71$^+$, is G_{ix}^-; we would attribute this to the fact that the type-specific determinants detected in the G_{ix} cytotoxic assay are lacking on the B6 gp69/71$^+$. By this explanation, thymocytes of $B6_{G_{ix}^+}$ mice, obtained by serial backcrosses between $129_{(G_{ix}^+)}$ and $B6_{(G_{ix}^-)}$, should contain genes coding for at least two species of gp69/71. In fact, we had previously shown that the concentration of gp69/71 in spleens of $B6_{G_{ix}^+}$ was greater than that of B6 and had attributed this to such a gene dosage effect.

Additional evidence supporting this hypothesis is that $129_{G_{ix}^+}$ and $B6_{G_{ix}^-}$ gp69/71$^+$ carry physically distinguishable gp69/71 components and that thymocytes of $B6_{G_{ix}^+}$ gp69/71$^+$ have a higher titer of gp69/71 than thymocytes of 129 or $B6_{G_{ix}^-}$ gp69/71, in agreement with our finding of elevated protein in the spleen of this strain (66).

It had earlier been suggested that the G_{ix} cell surface antigen was a cellular, not a viral, antigen. This recent finding that it is a constituent of the gp69/71 raised the question as to whether the G_{ix} section of the gp69/71 molecule is physically accessible to cytotoxic antibody when gp69/71 is present in the virion envelope, rather than on the cell surface. This now has been tested and it was found that intact murine virions do absorb the anti-G_{ix} reactivity of cytotoxic serum (42).

The occurrence of virus protein antigens as cell surface cytotoxic components has several biological implications. One is in relation to autoimmune disease. The genome of these viruses is present in normal cells and constitutively expresses gp69/71, and there is evidence that this protein induces autogenous antibodies in many strains of mice (28). Thus, a serious consideration is the possibility that the expression of this viral glycoprotein is the basis for autoimmune diseases such as lupus erythematosis in NZB mice (76). Another is the cellular response to oncogenesis. If genes for a transforming protein are closely linked to the gp69/71, as is suggested by work described below, then induction of oncogenesis may be accompanied by induction of gp69/71. The presence of this "foreign" antigen on cell surfaces could then provide a mechanism for cell killing by cytotoxic antibodies.

7. Involvement of gp69/71 in the Glomerulonephritis of New Zealand mice   The concentration of gp69/71 in the spleen of New Zealand mice (NZB, NZW, B/W$_{F_1}$, and W/B$_{F_1}$) is 10-fold greater than that found in spleen extracts of high leukemia mice and 1,000-fold greater than that found in BALB mice (76). The gp69/71 is also the main viral protein deposited in the diseased kidneys of mice, and the glomerular site and extent of deposition are related to severity of the glomerulonephritis. These findings suggest that the pathogenesis of immune complex glomerulonephritis in mice is in some manner related to the expression of the viral envelope glycoproteins and the host immune response to this protein.

C. Characterization of the Major Structural Protein (p30)

1. Chemical Properties As the major structural component of the virion, constituting 10–20% of the total protein of the virion, the p30 protein is being extensively studied. Structural analysis has shown that the p30 proteins of several mammalian type C viruses have a high degree of overall sequence homology (*46*). All examined, including cat, RD 114, and baboon, begin with the sequence prolylleucylarginyl (Pro-Leu-Arg), and have a conserved region from residues 11 to 24. Out of 24 residues of the NH_2-terminal sequence compared, only a single amino acid difference was found between six different mouse p30s.

2. Antigenic Properties The p30 protein contains both group and interspecies antigenic determinants (*20, 22, 23*). By radioimmunoassay, we have shown the presence of a weak fraction of type-specific determinants (*59*).

This protein, because of the strong interspecies reactivity, has proved extremely valuable for examination of the relatedness of different viruses. In a detailed study of these comparisons, the relatedness of antigenic determinants of purified p30 proteins of the murine, feline, RD 114/baboon, and woolly monkey/gibbon ape groups of RNA tumor viruses was examined by competition radioimmunoassay (*64*). The cross-reactive (interspecies) antigens of every two viruses were selectively examined by precipitating the purified ^{125}I-labeled protein with antiserum against each of the other proteins. The extent to which these shared determinants were common to the other viruses was then tested by the effectiveness of the proteins of each virus to compete for antibody binding. Several classes of interspecies determinants were distinguished: those common to two of the groups of viruses, others to three, and some to all four. Moreover, an even greater variety of interspecies determinants was indicated by differences in the affinity of the individual proteins for antibody binding, supporting the hypothesis that there are at least several, if not many, different interspecies determinants with a broad spectrum of antigenic cross-reactivity. These studies suggest that the murine and feline viruses are closely related because they contain cross-reactive antigenic determinants not shared with the other viruses, that the feline virus is more closely related to the woolly monkey virus than to RD 114, and that the RD 114 and woolly monkey viruses retain interspecies determinants shared relatively equally with each of the other viruses.

These findings have immediate importance in assays for the characterization of virus isolates or for the detection of viral gene expression in different animal species, including human. It is obvious that for the analysis of proteins of unknown viruses a procedure that is equally sensitive for all type C viruses is required to determine the concentration of the viral protein. The three most applicable assays for such an analysis are the ^{125}I-labeled murine p30 or ^{125}I-labeled feline p27: anti-RD 114 p28 serum system and the ^{125}I-labeled woolly monkey virus p28: anti-RD 114 p28 serum system. With either of these there is less than 10-fold difference in the affinity of the different viral proteins for the interspecies antibodies selected for in the assay system. With all other interspecies assay systems tested, the range of affinities of the different proteins is so great that they cannot be used to measure an unknown protein.

3. Evidence that p30 is Virus Coded   As described above for gp69/71, the analysis of Rauscher virus propagated in mouse, rat, or human cells by the homologous competition radioimmunoassay demonstrated that the antigenic determinants of the protein were virus-specific, irrespective of the host cell, thus providing evidence that this protein is virus coded.

D.   Characterization of the p15 Protein

1. Chemical Properties   A variable number of small molecular weight polypeptides of different sizes are found associated with the mammalian RNA tumor viruses (Figure 1). As yet, the chemical relatedness of these different polypeptides is largely unknown. It appears that the variation from one virus to another is so great that few, if any, generalizations are possible until a sufficient number of these proteins are purified and characterized. We have succeeded in purifying one of these proteins found in Rauscher murine leukemia virus that has an apparent molecular weight of 15,000 as determined by polyacrylamide gel electrophoresis in sodium dodecyl sulfate. As described below, the antigenic determinant of this protein (and thus presumably its amino acid composition) are highly type-specific. Thus it can be expected that the analogous protein of other viruses will also be distinctive and may not have the same size.

2. Antigenic Characterization   The bulk of the antigenic determinants of the Rauscher MuLV p15 are type- or subgroup-specific (63). The major antigenic reactivity of the protein was specific to Rauscher and Friend viruses and, to a lesser extent, to Moloney virus. Other murine viruses, Kirsten or AKR, as well as other species of viruses, FeLV or RD 114, showed little or no competition, indicating that at least 80–90% of the antibodies were directed to type-specific determinants. Group and interspecies determinants were also detected by use of the appropriate assay systems, but showed relatively minor reactivity.

3. Evidence that p15 is Virus Coded   The strong type-specificity of the antigenic determinants of the p15 protein is by itself virtual proof that this protein is virus coded. Nevertheless, as described above for the gp69/71 and p30 proteins, the antigenic determinants of p15 of Rauscher virus grown in mouse, rat, and human cells were compared by the competition radioimmunoassay and found to be identical.

4. Expression as FMR Cell Surface Antigen   Leukemia cells produced by infection with Friend, Moloney, or Rauscher virus induce cytotoxic antibodies that are cross-reactive with this group of infected cells (44). The FMR antigen is also found in disrupted virions of the subgroup of viruses (34). So as to define the specific identity of the FMR antigen, fractions from our purification procedure were assayed by Friedman and Lilly for an activity that blocked the cytotoxic antibodies in the FMR assay. It was found that the FMR antigen of Rauscher MuLV purified with the p15 protein and that monospecific antibodies to the p15 protein are cytotoxic in the FMR assay. It thus appears that the molecular species identified as the FMR antigen is the p15 protein.

E.   Translational Precursor Proteins and Genetic Linkage Groups

Synthesis of proteins of type C RNA tumor viruses, as of some other eukaryotic cell RNA viruses, occurs in the form of precursor polyproteins that are subsequently specifically cleaved to yield the mature viral proteins (16). Analysis of these precursor or polyproteins allows a unique opportunity to analyze the structural linkage relationships of the individual viral proteins. Such studies have been carried out utilizing monospecific antisera directed against the Rauscher virus gp69/71, p30, and p15 proteins, utilizing pulse-labeling and pulse-chase techniques, followed by immunoprecipitation and polyacrylamide gel electrophoresis of the viral protein (Figure 3)

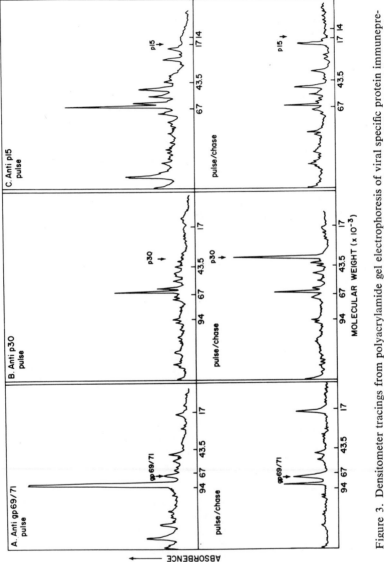

Figure 3. Densitometer tracings from polyacrylamide gel electrophoresis of viral specific protein immunepre-cipitates. Rauscher virus infected NRK cells were pulse labeled for 10 min with [^{35}S]methionine. or pulse labeled 10 min followed by 4 hr chase. (*A*) anti-gp69/71 serum immuneprecipitates; (*B*) anti-p30 serum immuneprecipitates; (*C*) anti-p15 serum immuneprecipitates.

The major envelope glycoprotein, gp69/71, was found to be a cleavage product of a 90,000-dalton precursor. Labeling experiments show that this 90,000-dalton precursor is also a glycoprotein. When labeling is performed in the presence of a 2-deoxy-D-glucose, an inhibitor of glycosylation, there is a nonglycosylated polypeptide of about 70,000 daltons that appears to be nonspecifically degraded. This suggests that the carbohydrate side chains of the glycoprotein play a role in specifying the precursor cleavage site and in protecting this virus protein from proteolytic degradation.

The p30 and p15 proteins were both found to be included in a 65,000-dalton precursor protein. It thus appears that these two virion proteins are closely linked in the viral genome.

We have also detected a possible precursor protein that appears to contain the antigenic determinants of all three virion proteins studied: gp69/71, p30, and p15. This polypeptide has a molecular weight of greater than 300,000 and is large enough to be the complete translation product of a 35 S Rauscher virus RNA genomic subunit. Thus far it has been found in much lower concentration than the 90,000- and 65,000-dalton precursors, indicating either that it is processed very rapidly or that the smaller proteins may be synthesized independently.

These data support a model that has the virus genome first translated as a polypeptide with a molecular weight of greater than 300,000 or as smaller precursor polyproteins (Figure 4). These

Provirus, 3 to 4 x 10^6 daltons

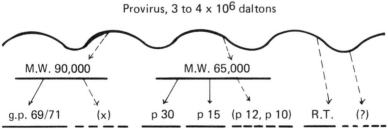

Figure 4. A model for post-translational processing of type C virus proteins. Evidence has been obtained for the synthesis of high molecular weight viral precursor proteins. One, a 90,000-dalton polypeptide, contains the gp69/71 proteins. There remains an additional 20,000 daltons of protein (X), which could possibly be an additional viral protein. A second intermediate precursor of 65,000 daltons contains the p30 and p15 proteins. The additional cleavage product of this precursor could possibly contain the small structural proteins p12 and p10. At least one additional cleavage product is required to yield the reverse transcriptase enzyme or other as yet unknown proteins.

possibly early cleavage products or primary precursors are a 90,000-dalton precursor containing the gp69/71 protein and a 65,000-dalton precursor containing the p30 and p15 proteins. Both of the intermediate-sized precursors could contain viral proteins in addition to those proteins we have studied. There must, in addition, be other cleavage products yielding the reverse transcriptase and possibly other yet unrecognized proteins.

III. GENE EXPRESSION OF DEFECTIVE SARCOMA VIRUSES

Another approach to the structure and organization of the viral genome is by the isolation and characterization of virus mutants. Of particular interest are the mammalian sarcoma viruses. These viruses, with one possible exception, are all defective for replication; synthesis of infectious progeny by sarcoma virus transformants has been found only upon concomitant infection with a helper leukemia virus (4). The nature of the defectiveness of sarcoma viruses differs among the isolates studied. Currently there are two classes of sarcoma viruses: (1) Those that lack any evidence of virus particle formation; cells infected by these viruses, designated as nonproducer cells, have not been found to synthesize a detectable level of any viral protein, although they possess a rescuable sarcoma virus genome and viral-specific mRNA (7, 26, 54, 69, 70). (2) Those that direct the synthesis of viral structural proteins; cells infected by such viruses, S^+L^-, HTG-1, and WSV-NRK, contain "viral gs antigen" and in some cases noninfectious viral particles are detected (5, 18, 54).

Recently, we found that infection of normal rat kidney cells (NRK) with the Kirsten murine sarcoma and leukemia virus complex at limiting dilution gave rise at equal frequency to two classes of nonproductively transformed cells; cells that contained gp69/71 at a concentration equal to that of transformed cells which produce virus and transformed cells that did not contain a detectable concentration (less than 0.1–1.0 ng of viral protein per mg of total cell protein) of either the major structural protein, p30, or the viral envelope glycopeptide gp69/71 (8). The expression of the viral envelope protein in the transformed cells can be explained in several ways. The primary consideration is that there is a close linkage of the sarcoma and glycoprotein genes in this defective-envelope–positive-sarcoma virus such that they are jointly integrated and expressed.

Another possibility is that the glycoprotein expressed is that of an NRK endogenous virus, because it is commonly found that transformation itself may lead to the induction of the endogenous viral genome. However, this alternative was not supported by the previous immunochemical studies of the envelope protein (*8*). In addition, it is at least theoretically possible that the infecting virus contained a high concentration of a defective leukemia virus ($p30^-$ $gp69/71^+$), and that the envelope-positive transformed cells resulted from simultaneous infection by this and a defective sarcoma virus, even though the cells were infected with a limiting dilution of virus. These alternatives have now been examined in two ways, by the interference properties of the infected cells and by rescue of the sarcoma virus genome.

Interference, the resistance of a virus-infected cell to superinfection with the same or a closely related virus, has been shown to be a property of the viral envelope glycopeptides. For this reason we have analyzed the interference properties of Kirsten transformed nonproducer cells in order to distinguish, by the pattern of interference murine, endogenous rat and woolly monkey virus. In these experiments Kirsten transformed, cloned, nonproducer cell lines were superinfected with murine and primate viruses and the efficiency of infection measured by the titer of rescued sarcoma virus. It was found that envelope-positive clones were resistant to superinfection with either of the two strains of murine viruses tested, whereas envelope-negative cells were readily infected. In contrast, both envelope-positive and envelope-negative clones were rescuable upon superinfection with a woolly monkey virus (WoLV). Due to the reported limited infectivity of rat endogenous virus, rescue experiments were also performed by cocultivation; no significant difference in the rescuability of the two cell types by VNRK or WoLV was observed. Differential rescue could even be demonstrated in cocultivation experiments where three log lower titers of focus-forming virus were rescued from expressor cells by cocultivation with Rauscher-producing cells. As a control for these studies, to demonstrate that absence of sarcoma genome rescue by murine viruses from the envelope-positive cells could be attributed to interference and not some other block in viral replication, Sendai virus mediated cell fusion was carried out. This was based upon earlier studies of viral interference that indicated that the absorption and penetration steps of viral replication were involved in restriction of avian viruses in nonpermissive cells and these steps could be bypassed with cell fusion techniques. After cell fusion of Kirsten transformed cells to Rauscher virus-producing NRK cells, the titer of rescued sarcoma virus was the same for envelope-positive and envelope-negative cells, clearly demonstrating that the inability of murine viruses to rescue expressor cells can be bypassed by cell fusion. Cocultivation under the same conditions, but in the absence of inactivated Sendai virus, had little effect upon the yield of sarcoma virus from expressor cells.

The possible linkage of envelope and sarcoma genes was also investigated by rescue with woolly monkey virus. Both envelope-positive and negative cells were superinfected with woolly monkey virus and the rescued sarcoma virus in the tissue culture fluids were diluted and used to infect NRK cells. Random foci were isolated from plates containing less than 10 foci, grown to mass culture, and characterized by radioimmunoassay for the murine gp69/71 antigenic determinants. Ten of 14 transformed cell lines obtained by rescue of envelope-positive cells demonstrated gp69/71 as well as transformation genes. In contrast, all 15 clones derived from virus rescued from envelope-negative cells had no detectable gp69/71.

Additional information about the proteins coded for by these defective sarcoma viruses has been obtained by characterization of the viral precursor polyproteins. Polypeptides labeled during a 10-min pulse with [^{35}S]methionine were precipitated with mono-specific antisera against purified Rauscher gp69/71. A protein of approximately 90,000 daltons was present in envelope-positive NRK cells and not in envelope-negative Kirsten transformants. The size of the polypeptide precipitated with anti-gp69/71 was similar to that found in NRK cells producing Rauscher, MEV, or the Kirsten sarcoma leukemia complex. Thus it appears that the mRNA coding for the gp69/71 is the same in cells infected with infectious virus and the defective sarcoma virus.

The available evidence suggests that there is a defective KiMuSV that contains the genetic information for both murine gp69/71 and transformation functions and that they are closely linked. As yet, however, little is known of the organization of specific genes of mammalian type C RNA tumor viruses.

In this respect unravelling the genotype of mammalian sarcoma viruses is substantially more difficult because they do not replicate in the absence of helper virus. Also, the stability of sarcoma virus phenotypes despite the formation of pseudotypes with type C helper viruses, coupled with the failure to isolate helper-independent sarcoma virus recombinants at any reasonable frequency, suggests lengthy deletions or other significant changes in the organization of the genes in sarcoma viruses.

IV.   HOST CELL CONTROL OF GENE EXPRESSION

The genome of the murine leukemia virus is known to be an endogenous inheritable factor of normal cellular DNA, and viral genetic sequences can be found in normal cellular DNA. The expression of these viral genes is obviously controlled, as is that of any other cellular gene. Mice of the AKR, C58, PL, and a few other strains show a high incidence of spontaneous leukemia and begin to express infectious viruses in their tissues soon after birth. Mice of other strains are usually virus-free early in life and show a low incidence of spontaneous leukemia. These earlier studies of viral gene expression in mice have depended chiefly upon the synthesis of infectious virus or of particles containing reverse transcriptase. Because these types of assays depend upon the presence of all or most of the viral structural proteins, they do not provide evidence concerning the possible expression and regulation of individual viral proteins. Recently, in collaboration with Lilly we have made use of specific radioimmunoassays for individual viral gene products, the gp69/71 and p30, as a means to measure quantitatively the concentration of these proteins in tissues of mice regardless of whether virus was produced or not (Table 2) (*65, 66*).

A.   High Leukemic Mouse Strains and Crosses

Mice of the high leukemia strains show high concentrations of both p30 and gp69/71 in their tissues at concentrations of the same ratio as found in the virions. At this time, it is unknown why the "V" genes of the high-incidence strains are more readily expressed than those of other strains. An approach to this important problem has been initiated by analysis of crosses between different strains. F_1 crosses of AKR with low leukemic C57L mice showed the high AKR concentration of p30 and gp69/71, rather than the low C57L levels. This finding is consistent with the fact that virus expression is dominant in this cross (*49*). Although C57L mice show no

Table 2. Expression of MuLV p30 and gp69/71 in spleens of inbred mice

Strain	p30	gp69/71
	(ng viral protein per mg spleen protein[a])	
High leukemia		
AKR	105 ± 13 (5)	60 ± 20 (2)
C58/J	210	100
PL/J	75 ± 9 (4)	48 ± 3 (4)
Low leukemia		
BALB/c	4 ± 2 (3)	1 ± 0 (2)
BALB/c-nu/nu[b]	5	10
BALB/c-+/nu[b]	5	1
BALB · B	6 ± 1 (2)	0.6 ± 0.1 (6)
BALB · K	5	1
C57L	6 ± 1.8 (7)	6 ± 2 (2)
B10 (C57BL/Sn)	1	11
B10 · BR	80	10
B10 · A	1	12
B10 · D2new	0.5	10
B10 · A(2R)	3	20
B6 (C57BL/6)	20	25
B6-G_{ix}^{+c}	23 ± 0 (2)	100 ± 0 (2)
B6-H-2^k	1	20
DBA/2	20 ± 3 (4)	175 ± 25 (4)
DBA/2-Fv-1[b]	85 ± 6 (5)	55 ± 9 (5)
129[c]	6 ± 1 (3)	10 ± 1 (3)
129-G_{ix}^{-c}	0.1 ± 0 (3)	1.0 ± 0 (3)
P/J	1	10
A	7	15
RF/J	6	1
F_1 hybrids		
C57L × AKR	133 ± 33 (3)	50
BALB/c × AKR	32	4
BALB · B × AKR	40	3
BALB/c × DBA/2	11 ± 1 (5)	3 ± 0.4 (5)
B10 × B10 · BR	181 ± 5 (3)	40 ± 0 (3)
DBA/2 × 129-G_{ix}^{-c}	10	25
129-G_{ix}^- × AKR[c]	80	25

Mice identified with /J were obtained from the Jackson Laboratory.

[a]Values represent either single determinations with a pool of three to four spleens or the mean (± SEM) values of determinations with individual spleen extracts; the number in parentheses is the number of extracts examined.

[b]Mice obtained by the courtesy of Dr. Seung-il Shin, Albert Einstein College of Medicine.

[c]Mice obtained by the courtesy of Dr. Elisabeth Stockert, Sloan-Kettering Institute.

infectious MuLV in their tissues, their $Fv-1^n$ genotype is permissive for the expression of N-tropic AKR virus. In contrast, F_1 crosses of AKR with low leukemia BALB/c mice showed reduced expression of both p30 and especially gp69/71 in comparison with their AKR parents. Thus some dominant genetic control factor is operative in the BALB strain. One possibility is that the suppression in these hybrids is due to the dominant $Fv-1^b$ allele inherited from the BALB/c parent. However, this does not exclude the possibility of other regulatory functions of the BALB parent, and further analysis of segregation of the F_2 offspring should be carried out.

B. DBA/2 and Related Mice

DBA/2 mice, which show only a low incidence of spontaneous leukemia, nevertheless show moderate amounts of p30 and quite high levels of gp69/71. In contrast, mice of the partially congenic DBA/2-$Fv-1^b$ strain show increased levels of p30 and decreased levels of gp69/71 in comparison with DBA/2 strain mice. Since the $Fv-1$ gene is known to play a significant regulatory role in the expression of endogenous MuLV, it may be speculated that this gene might influence the expression of MuLV-related proteins and that the DBA/2 genome includes a B-tropic "V" gene that is more readily expressed in permissive $Fv-1^b$ than in restrictive $Fv-1^n$ cells.

C. B10 Congenic Mice

The $H-2$ region of chromosome 17 (linkage group IX) of the mouse includes a gene or genes of importance in the regulation of susceptibility to viral leukemogenesis. For this reason the well-known $H-2$-congenic strains of the C57BL/10Sn (B10) background, B10.BR ($H-2^k$), B10 ($H-2^b$), B10.A ($H-2^a$), B10.D2 ($H-2^d$), and B10/A ($H-2^h$) have been examined for levels of p30 and of gp69/71. No significant effect on viral protein concentration in spleen cells that could be attributed to the $H-2$ genes was detected.

D. BALB/c Mice

Mice of the low leukemia BALB/c strain show low but significant levels of p30, but these mice show at most trace amounts of gp69/71 activity. This strain is, in this respect, the opposite of B10, which showed low p30. The virtual absence of gp69/71 is a dominant trait, for F_1 crosses of BALB/c with high-gp69/71 mice (AKR, DBA/2) also show strongly suppressed levels of gp69/71. Since suppression of gp69/71 is the dominant trait, it is reasonable to suppose that one or more regulatory genes are the basis of this phenomenon.

Mice of the congenic BALB/c subline carrying the *nude* gene have also been examined. *Nude* mice lack most immunologic capacities for which T cells are a requirement (*51*). Normal ($+/+$ or $+/nu$) littermates of *nude* mice of this strain were indistinguishable from BALB/c mice of their own colony, but *nude* homozygotes (*nu/nu*) showed a dramatic increase in gp69/71 activity.

Our interpretation of these findings is that BALB/c mice possess one or more structural genes for the gp69/71 molecule, but the expression of this substance is specifically repressed by the action of a dominant regulatory gene also carried by these mice. This suppression of gp69/71 may be mediated by an immunologic mechanism of some sort, since in *nude* mice, which have a basic defect in their immunologic capacity, this suppression is not seen.

V. RNA TUMOR VIRUS GENE EXPRESSION IN HUMAN TISSUE

Animal model systems indicate a possible relatedness of type C viruses to neoplasia, autoimmune diseases, and central nervous system diseases (*2, 27, 36*). These diseases of inbred strains of mice are associated with higher tissue concentrations of infectious virus and viral proteins. However, there is little evidence that these viruses infect and cause disease in man.

As an extension of the work described above, utilizing purified proteins from a variety of known RNA tumor viruses and immuno-chemical techniques, we recently demonstrated the presence of a viral p30 protein in human tissues (*60*). For these studies screening of tissues was carried out by use of a heterologous assay system of ^{125}I-labeled Rauscher murine virus p30 antigen and anti-RD 114 virus serum, because this system was found to detect a class of interspecies determinants common to murine, feline, and primate viruses. A competitor with the same apparent affinity for antibody binding as that of purified viral core proteins was found in relatively high concentrations in tissues from patients with systemic lupus erythematosis, in some neoplastic tissues, and also in normal human tissues. This competitor from a lupus spleen chromatographed on phosphocellulose and showed size fractionation during gel filtration similar to known p27 to p30 viral proteins. An immunologically reactive protein was also demonstrated by immunodiffusion and by immunoprecipitation of ^{125}I-labeled human protein with anti-RD 114 p28 serum. Analysis of these partially purified human competitor fractions of human tissues with homologous assay systems of viral core proteins and corresponding antisera showed that almost all, including those of the normal tissue extracts, reacted chiefly with both the RD 114 and woolly monkey species. In the case of one extract of a lupus tissue, the principle reactivity was in the murine system.

VI. DISCUSSION

The primary objectives of the studies described here are the identification of type C virus gene products, their isolation and characterization, and the use of these proteins as probes for analysis of the organization and function of the viral genome.

One of the important questions that may be addressed with current findings concerns the control of expression of individual viral genes: Is control coordinated so that all of the genes are expressed concomitantly as in the synthesis of virions, or is there independent control of transcription, translation, or degradation of individual genes or gene products? The available evidence suggests that individual genes or groups of genes may be independently expressed and that in some cases specific viral gene products may be synthesized as products of apparently normal cells. However, as yet the data are not conclusive. Independent control of expression of gene products is immediately suggested by the differences in relative concentrations of virion proteins. The most notable example of this is the reverse transcriptase, which is present in much lower concentration, 1% or less, than other structural proteins. However, there remains the possibility that the enzyme is synthesized at a concentration comparable to the other proteins but is degraded more rapidly or is not all packaged in the virion. These questions require use of specific antiserum to analyze the cellular concentration of the enzyme and its rate of synthesis by pulse-labeling and pulse-chase experiments. With respect to other proteins, the animal tissue concentration of gp69/71 and p30 vary markedly from one species to another, as shown here. The interpretation of these experiments is limited, however, because it is not known whether the concentration of a protein is the function of genome transcription, mRNA translation, or protein degradation. Moreover, there is also the possibility that synthesis of any given protein results from a partial or defective genome capable of synthesizing only one or another protein and is not the result of independent control of specific viral genes. Additional data on this topic are being provided by the use of pulse-labeling techniques to analyze the synthesis of high molecular weight viral precursor proteins. Current findings suggest the presence of at least three protein linkage groups, one containing the envelope glycoprotein, another the p30 and p15 and with avian viruses other small molecular weight proteins, and, by necessity, one containing the reverse transcriptase. It remains to be determined whether each of these is derived from a single precursor corresponding to the entire genome, which then would require control mechanisms at the translational or degrading levels, or whether each may come from a separate mRNA, which would permit transcriptional control.

The application of these techniques to the analysis of human tissues indicates that type C virus gene expression is a feature of human cells as well. Viral proteins were detected in each of several *normal* human tissues tested, suggesting either the presence of endogenous viral genes, as occurs in other species, or widespread infection by exogenous viruses. In almost every case characterization of the protein in the positive tissues showed that proteins analogous to those of both the woolly monkey/gibbon ape group and the baboon/RD 114 group of viruses were detected. Thus humans appear to carry both of the currently known groups of primate RNA tumor viruses, either as endogenous or infective viruses. The findings of related viruses in new world and old world monkeys and humans, and in cats, baboons, and humans, indicate that there is wide species distribution. No evidence was found for a unique "human" group of RNA tumor virus. Such a virus, if it exists, is rare and perhaps should not be expected because of the close evolutionary relatedness of humans to other primates. Of the limited number of tissues examined there were no significant differences in the concentrations of viral proteins in normal as compared to malignant tissues. This comparison requires extensive further analysis. The importance of the point is that the concentration of viral protein as a measurement of virus or viral gene products may be indicative of malignancy arising as a viral infectious process, as compared to disease induced in some other manner. With mice it is known that tumors induced by chemical or physical agents may have a normal concentration of viral proteins, whereas tumors arising from infection by virus have an elevated concentration. As yet, our results do not support the concept that the human tumors examined arose as a result of virus infection. One apparent correlation was a markedly elevated level of viral protein in tissues of patients with systemic lupus erythematosus, an autoimmune disease. A possible role of RNA tumor viruses in the etiology of this disease has previously been suggested by the close correlation in mice of the occurrence and severity of a lupus syndrome with the expression of an endogenous RNA tumor virus (76).

ACKNOWLEDGMENT

We are indebted to Jack Gruber and the Office of Program Resources and Logistics, National Cancer Institute, through whose courtesy we were provided with the Rauscher murine virus used in this investigation.

LITERATURE CITED

1. Abrell, J. W. and R. C. Gallo (1973). Purification, characterization, and comparison of the DNA polymerases from two primate RNA tumor viruses. J. Virol. 12:431–439.
2. Andrews, J. M. and M. B. Gardner (1974). Lower motor neuron degeneration associated with type-C RNA virus infection in mice: Neuropathological features. J. Neuropathol. Exp. Neurol. 33: 285–296.
3. August, J. T., D. P. Bolognesi, E. Fleissner, R. V. Gilden, and R. C. Nowinski (1974). A proposed nomenclature for the virion protein of oncogenic RNA viruses. Virology 60:595–601.
4. Ball, J. K., J. A. McCarter, and S. M. Sunderland (1973). Evidence of helper independent murine sarcoma virus. I. Segregation of replication-defective and transformation-defective viruses. Virology 56:264–268.
5. Bassin, R. H., L. A. Phillips, M. J. Kramer, D. K. Haepala, P. T. Peebles, S. Nomura, and P. J. Fischinger (1971). Transformation of mouse 3T3 cells by murine sarcoma virus: Release of virus-like particle in the absence of replicating murine leukemia helper virus. Proc. Nat. Acad. Sci. U.S.A. 68:1520–1524.
6. Bellamy, A. R., S. C. Gillies, and J. D. Harvey (1974). Molecular weights of two oncornavirus genomes: Deprivation from particle molecular weights and RNA content. J. Virol. 14:1388–1393.
7. Benveniste, R. E., G. J. Todaro, E. M. Scolnick, and W. P. Parks (1973). Partial transcription of murine type-C viral genomes in BALB/c cell lines. J. Virol. 12:711–720.

8. Bilello, J. A., M. Strand, and J. T. August (1974). Murine sarcoma virus gene expression: Transformants which express viral envelope glycoprotein in the absence of the major internal protein and infectious particles. Proc. Nat. Acad. Sci. U.S.A. 71:3234–3238.
9. Bolognesi, D. P. (1974) Structural components of RNA tumor viruses. *In: Advances in Virus Research,* F. G. Bang, Ed., Vol. 19, pp. 315–359. Academic Press, New York.
10. Boyse, E. A. and D. Bennett (1974). Differentiation and the cell surface: Illustration from work with T cells and sperm. *In:* G. M. Edelman (ed.), *Cellular Selection and Regulation in the Immune Response.* Society of General Physiological Series, Vol. 29, p. 155. Raven Press, New York.
11. Chattopadhyay, S. K., D. R. Lowy, N. M. Teich, A. S. Levine, and W. P. Rowe (1974). Qualitative and quantitative studies of AKR-type murine leukemia virus sequences in mouse DNA. Cold Spring Harbor Symp. Quant. Biol., 39:1085–1101.
12. Delius, H., P. H. Duesberg, and W. F. Mangel (1974). Electron microscope measurements of rous sarcoma virus RNA. Cold Spring Harbor Symp. Quant. Biol. (2), 39:835–843.
13. Del Villano, B. C., B. Nave, B. P. Croker, R. A. Lerner, and F. J. Dixon (1975). The oncornavirus glycoprotein gp69/71: A constitutent of the surface of normal and malignant thymocytes. J. Exp. Med. 141:172–187.
14. Duesberg, P. H., G. S. Martin, and P. K. Vogt (1970). Glycoprotein components of avian and murine RNA tumor viruses. Virology 41:631–646.
15. Duesberg, P., P. K. Vogt, K. Beemon, and M. Lai (1974). Avian RNA tumor viruses: Mechanism of recombination and complexity of the genome. Cold Spring Harbor Symp. Quant. Biol. (2), 39:847–857.
16. Eisenman, R., V. M. Vogt, and H. Diggelmann (1974). Synthesis of avian RNA tumor virus structural proteins. Cold Spring Harbor Symp. Quant. Biol. (2), 39:1067–1075.
17. Fleissner, E. (1971). Chromatographic separation and antigenic analysis of proteins of the oncornaviruses. I. Avian leukemia-sarcoma viruses. J. Virol. 8:778–785.
18. Gazdar, A. F., L. A. Phillips, P. S. Sarma, P. T. Peebles, and H. C. Chopra (1971). Presence of sarcoma genome in a "non-infectious" mammalian virus. Nature New Biol. 234:69–72.
19. Geering, G., T. Aoki, and L. J. Old (1970). Shared viral antigen of mammalian leukemia viruses. Nature (London) 226:265–266.
20. Geering, G., W. D. Hardy, Jr., L. J. Old, E. de Harven, and R. S. Brodey (1968). Shared group-specific antigen of murine and feline leukemia viruses. Virology 36:678–707.
21. Gerard, G. F. and D. P. Grandgenett (1975). Purification and characterization of the DNA polymerase and RNase H activities in Moloney murine sarcoma-leukemia virus. J. Virol. 15:785–797.

22. Gilden, R. V., S. Oroszlan, and R. J. Huebner (1971). Coexistence of intraspecies and intraspecies-specific antigenic determinants on the major structural polypeptide of mammalian C-type viruses. Nature New Biol. 231:107–108.

23. Gregoriades, A. and L. J. Old (1969). Isolation and some characteristics of a group-specific antigen of the murine leukemia viruses. Virology 37:189–202.

24. Gross, L. (1970). *Oncogenic Viruses,* 2nd ed., Pergamon Press, Oxford, England.

25. Hanafusa, T., H. Hanafusa, T. Miyamoto, and E. Fleissner (1972). Existence and expression of tumor virus genes in chick embryo cells. Virology 47:475.

26. Huebner, R. J., J. W. Hartley, W. P. Rowe, W. T. Lane, and W. J. Capps (1966). Rescue of the defective genome of Moloney sarcoma virus from a noninfectious hamster tumor and the production of pseudotype sarcoma viruses with various leukemia viruses. Proc. Nat. Acad. Sci. U.S.A. 56:1164–1169.

27. Huebner, R. J. and G. J. Todaro (1969). Oncogenes of RNA tumor viruses as determinants of cancer. Proc. Nat. Acad. Sci. U.S.A. 64:1087–1094.

28. Ihle, J. N., M. G. Hanna, Jr., L. E. Roberson, and F. T. Kenney (1974). Autogenous immunity to endogenous RNA tumor virus: Identification of antibody reactivity to select viral antigens. J. Exp. Med. 139:1568–1581.

29. Ikeda, H., T. Pincus, T. Yoshiki, M. Strand, J. T. August, E. A. Boyse, and R. C. Mellors (1974). Biological expression of antigenic determinants of murine leukemia virus protein gp69/71 and p30. J. Virol. 14:1274–1280.

30. Kaplan, H. S. (1967). On the natural history of the murine leukemias: Presidential address. Cancer Res. 27:1325.

31. Kawai, S. and H. Hanafusa (1971). The effects of reciprocal changes in temperature on the transformed state of cells infected with a Rous sarcoma virus mutant. Virology 46:470–479.

32. Kennel, S. J., B. C. Del Villano, R. L. Levy, and R. A. Lerner (1973). Properties of an oncornavirus glycoprotein: Evidence for its presence on the surface of virions and infected cells. Virology 55:464–475.

33. Kung, H. J., J. M. Bailey, N. Davidson, P. K. Vogt, M. O. Nicolson, and R. M. McAllister (1974). Electron microscope studies of tumor vrius RNA. Cold Spring Harbor Symp. Quant. Biol. (2), 39:827–834.

34. Lilly, F. and R. Steeves (1974). Antigens of murine leukemia viruses. Biochem. Biophys. Acta (CR) 355:105.

35. Linial, M. and W. S. Mason (1973). Characterization of two conditional early mutants of Rous sarcoma virus. Virology 53:258–273.

36. Mellors, R. C. (1966). Autoimmune and immunoproliferative diseases in NZB mice and hybrids. Int. Rev. Exp. Path. 5:217.

37. Moelling, K. (1974). Characterization of reverse transcriptase and RNase H from Friend murine leukemia virus. Virology 62:46–59.
38. Moennig, V., H. Frank, G. Hunsmann, I. Schnieider, and W. Schafer (1974). Properties of mouse leukemia viruses VII. The major viral glycoprotein of Friend leukemia virus. Isolation and physicochemical properties. Virology 61:100–111.
39. Moroni, C. (1972). Structural proteins of Rauscher leukemia virus and Harvey sarcoma virus. Virology 47:1–7.
40. Nowinski, R. C., E. Fleissner, N. H. Sarkar, and T. Aoki (1972). Chromatographic separation and antigenic analysis of proteins of the oncornaviruses. H. Mammalian leukemia-sarcoma viruses. J. Virol. 9:359–366.
41. Nowinski, R. C. and E. D. Peters (1973). Cell surface antigens associated with murine leukemia virus: Definition of the G_L and G_T antigenic systems. J. Virol. 12:1104.
42. Obata, Y., H. Ikeda, E. Stockert, and E. A. Boyse (1975). Relation of G_{ix} antigen of thymocytes to envelope glycoprotein of murine leukemia virus. J. Exp. Med. 141:188–197.
43. Old, L. J. and E. A. Boyse (1973). Current enigmas in cancer research. Harvey Lectures 67:273.
44. Old, L. J., E. A. Boyse, and E. Stockert (1964). Typing of mouse leukemias by serological methods. Nature 201:777.
45. Oroszlan, S., D. Bova, M. H. M. White, R. Toni, C. Foremen, and R. V. Gilden (1972). Purification and immunological characterization of the major internal protein of the RD 114 virus. Proc. Nat. Acad. Sci. U.S.A. 69:1211–1215.
46. Oroszlan, S., T. Copeland, M. R. Summers, G. Smythers, and R. V. Gilden (1975). Amino acid sequence homology of mammalian type-C RNA virus major internal protein. J. Biol. Chem. 52:6232–6239.
47. Oskarsson, M. K., W. G. Robey, C. L. Harris, P. J. Fischinger, D. K Haapala, and G. F. Vande Woude (1975). A p60 polypeptide in the feline leukemia virus pseudotype of Moloney sarcoma virus with murine leukemia virus p30 antigenic determinants. Proc. Nat. Acad. Sci. U.S.A. 72:2380–2384.
48. Parks, W. P., M. C. Noon, R. Gilden, and E. M. Scolnick (1975). Serological studies with low-molecular-weight polypeptides from the Moloney strain of murine leukemia virus. J. Virol. 15:1385–1395.
49. Rowe, W. P. (1972). Studies of genetic transmission of murine leukemia virus by AKR mice. I. Crosses with $Fv-1^n$ strains of mice. J. Exp. Med. 136:1272.
50. Rowe, W. P. (1973). Genetic factors in the natural history of murine leukemia virus infection: G. H. A. Clowes Memorial lecture. Cancer Res. 33:3061.
51. Rygaard, J. (1973). Thymus and self. Immunology of The Mouse Mutant Nude. F. A. D. L., Copenhagen.

52. Schafer, W., G. Hunsmann, V. Moennig, F. De Noronha, D. P. Bolognesi, R. W. Green, and G. Huper (1975). Polypeptides of mammalian oncornaviruses. II. Characterization of a murine leukemia virus polypeptide (p15) bearing interspecies reactivity. Virology 63:48–59.

53. Schafer, W., J. Lange, P. J. Fischinger, H. Frank, D. P. Bolognesi, and L. Pister (1972). Properties of mouse leukemia virus. II. Isolation of viral components. Virology 47:210–228.

54. Scollnick, E. M. and W. P. Parks (1973). Isolation and characterization of a primate sarcoma virus: Mechanism of rescue. Int. J. Cancer 12:138–147.

55. Steeves, R. A., M. Strand, and J. T. August (1974). Structural proteins of mammalian oncogenic RNA viruses: Murine leukemia virus neutralizations by antisera prepared against purified envelope glycoprotein. J. Virol. 14:187–189.

56. Stockert, E., L. J. Old, and E. A. Boyse (1971). The G_{ix} system. Cell surface allo-antigen associated with murine leukemia virus: Implications regarding chromosomal integration of the viral genomes. J. Exp. Med. 133:1334.

57. Stockert, E., H. Sato, K. Itakura, E. A. Boyse, L. J. Old, and J. J. Hutton (1972). Location of the second gene required for expression of the leukemia-associated mouse antigen G_{ix}. Science 178:862.

58. Strand, M. and J. T. August (1973). Structural proteins of oncogenic ribonucleic acid viruses. J. Biol. Chem. 248:5627–5633.

59. Strand, M. and J. T. August (1974a). Structural proteins of mammalian oncogenic RNA viruses: Multiple antigenic determinants of the major internal protein and envelope glycoprotein. J. Virol. 13:171–180.

60. Strand, M. and J. T. August (1974b). Type-C RNA virus gene expression in human tissue. J. Virol. 14:1584–1596.

61. Strand, M. and J. T. August (1974c). Structural proteins of RNA tumor viruses as probes for viral gene expression. Cold Spring Harbor Symp. Quant. Biol. 39:1109–1116.

62. Strand, M. and J. T. August (1974d). Purification and immunologic characterization of three interspecies proteins of mammalian C-type RNA tumor viruses. Cancer and Leukemia Viruses Proceedings of the U.S.A.–U.S.S.R. Symposium, 182–189.

63. Strand, M., R. Wilsnack, and J. T. August (1974e). Structural proteins of mammalian oncogenic RNA viruses: Immunological characterization of the p15 polypeptide of Rauscher murine virus. J. Virol. 14:1575–1583.

64. Strand, M. and J. T. August (1975). Structural proteins of mammalian RNA tumor viruses: Relatedness of the interspecies antigenic determinants of the major internal protein. J. Virol. 15:1332–1341.

65. Strand, M., F. Lilly, and J. T. August (1974a). Host control of endogenous murine leukemia virus gene expression: Concentra-

tions of viral proteins in high and low leukemia mouse strains. Proc. Nat. Acad. Sci. U.S.A. 71:3682–3686.

66. Strand, M., F. Lilly, and J. T. August (1974b). Genetic control of the expression of murine leukemia virus proteins in tissues of normal, young adult mice. Cold Spring Harbor Symp. Quant. Biol. 39:1117–1122.

67. Temin, H. M. (1974). Relationships among RNA tumor viruses and between RNA tumor viruses and cells: Implication for the origin of viruses, the evolution of vertebrates and cellular genetic systems. Ann. Rev. Gen. 8:155–178.

68. Todaro, G. J., R. E. Benveniste, R. Callahan, M. M. Lieber, and C. J. Sherr (1975). Endogenous primate and feline type-C viruses. Cold Spring Harbor Symp. Quant. Biol. 39:1159–1168.

69. Tronick, S. R., J. R. Stephenson, and S. A. Aaronson (1973). Immunological characterization of a low molecular weight polypeptide of murine leukemia virus. Virology 54:199–206.

70. Tsuchida, N., M. S. Robin, and M. Green (1972). Viral RNA subunits in cells transformed by RNA tumor viruses. Science 176: 1418–1419.

71. Tung, J. S., E. S. Vitetta, E. Fleissner, and E. Boyse (1975a). Biochemical evidence linking the G_{ix} thymocyte surface antigen to the gp69/71 envelope glycoprotein of murine leukemia virus. J. Exp. Med. 141:198–205.

72. Tung, J. S., E. Fleissner, E. S. Vitetta, and E. A. Boyse (1975b). Expression of MuLV envelope glycoprotein gp69/71 on mouse thymocytes: Evidence for two structural variants distinguished by presence versus absence of G_{ix} antigen. J. Exp. Med. 142:518–523.

73. Verma, I. M. (1975). Studies on reverse transcriptase of RNA tumor viruses. III. Properties of purified Moloney murine leukemia virus DNA polymerase and associated RNase H. J. Virol. 15:843–854.

74. Weissmann, C., J. T. Parsons, J. W. Coffin, L. Rymo, M. A. Billeter, and H. Hofstetter (1974). Studies on the structure and synthesis of Rous sarcoma virus RNA. Cold Spring Harbor Symp. Quant. Biol. 39:1043–1056.

75. Witte, O. N., I. L. Weissmann, and H. S. Kaplan (1973). Structural characteristics of some murine RNA tumor viruses studied by lactoperoxidase iodination. Proc. Nat. Acad. Sci. U.S.A. 70:36.

76. Yoshiki, T., R. C. Mellors, M. Strand, and J. T. August (1974). The viral envelope glycoprotein of murine leukemia virus and the pathogenesis of immune complex glomerulonephritis of New Zealand mice. J. Exp. Med. 140:1011.

CHAPTER 2

Type C Virogenes: Genetic Transfer and Interspecies Transfer

G. J. Todaro

I. TRANSMISSION OF VIROGENES

In the course of studies on the development of mouse cell lines in culture it was noted that certain spontaneously transformed cells began to release type C RNA tumor viruses (*1, 2, 14*). This finding, along with several other observations on the presence of viral specific antigens in the embryo of several mouse strains led to the hypothesis (virogene-oncogene hypothesis) that the information for the formation of such viruses might be transmitted genetically from parent to progeny along with other cellular genes (*7, 15*) (Table 1).

Activation of this normally repressed genetically transmitted type C virogene information, rather than infection from outside the animal, was proposed as the most common mechanism by which type C RNA tumor viruses are maintained in animal populations and produce naturally occurring cancers. Much subsequent experimental work supports this hypothesis, the most important being that "virus-free" cell lines (Table 2) derived from chicken, mouse, hamster, rat, pig, cat, and baboon tissues can begin to secrete typical complete type C viruses, either spontaneously or after treatment with chemical inducing agents. Co-cultivation with permissive cell lines from heterologous species has been needed to detect and to amplify virus production in several instances. In general, avian and mammalian cells in culture have been resistant to superinfection by their own endogenous type C viruses. The properties that charac-

Table 1. Implications of the virogene-oncogene hypothesis

Virogenes

1. All somatic cells of a species have DNA homologous to type C virus RNA of that species (virogenes).
2. Type C viruses derived from closely related species should have closely related specific antigens, e.g., gs antigens, polymerase, and their nucleic acid sequences should be more related to one another than are those viruses released by distantly related species (virogene evolution).

Oncogenes

3. The transformation-specific sequences of RNA tumor viruses should be present in normal cellular DNA (oncogenes).
4. Spontaneous, chemically induced, and viral-induced transformed cells and tumor cells should have RNA as well as DNA sequences homologous to the transforming specific sequences found in tumor viruses (oncogene expression).

Table 2. Species where a complete virogene is known to be present in normal cells

Chicken
Chinese hamster
Syrian hamster
Mouse *(Mus musculus)*
Mouse *(Mus caroli)*
Rat
Cat
Pig
Baboon

Table 3. Properties of endogenous type C virogenes

1. In the DNA of all somatic and germ cells of all the animals in a species.
2. Multiple related but not identical copies present in the cellular DNA, more than DNA from a heterologous cell that is actively producing virus.
3. Virus expression (RNA, gs antigen, polymerase, complete particles) under cellular control. Expressed in certain tissues at certain times during development.
4. Cells generally resistant to exogenous infection by the homologous endogenous virus.
5. Clonal lines either spontaneously or after induction are capable of releasing complete virion.

terize such endogenous mammalian type C viruses, the products of the genetically transmitted virogenes, are summarized in Table 3.

The endogenous type C virogenes are those sets of gene sequences that are an integral part of the host species' chromosomal DNA that code for the production of type C viruses. These genetically transmitted endogenous virogenes should be distinguished from type C viral DNA sequences that can be added to the animal's genome by "exogenous" viral infection and subsequent integration (provirus formation) (12). Endogenous type C virogenes should also be distinguished from those gene sequences not originally present in the genome, which are postulated to form by gene duplication and/or recombination during the lifetime of the animal through the mediation of the reverse transcriptase mechanism (protovirus formation) (3, 11, 13) (Table 4).

The sets of virogenes that a particular species possesses are normally repressed, but can be activated by a variety of intrinsic (genetic, hormonal) as well as extrinsic (radiation, chemical carcinogens, other infecting viruses) factors. As cellular genes, type C virogenes are subject to the pressures of mutation and selection; as such, closely related animal species would be expected to have closely related endogenous type C virogenes. What is unique about type C virogenes as distinguished from most other cellular genes, however, is that, at least in some species, they can give rise to the production of infectious type C virus particles. Since endogenous

Table 4. Major differences between virogene and protovirus models

Virogene	Protovirus
1. Complete copies present in germ cells and somatic cells.	1. Germ cells lack virus information. Generated in rare somatic cells by chance.
2. Genes maintained in population by normal cellular replication. Reverse transcriptase *not required.*	2. Reverse transcriptase plays essential role in generating new viruses.
3. Transformation results from activation of normally latent cellular genes associated with and/or part of the viral gene sequences.	3. Transformation results from the generation of new gene sequences by reverse transcription that do not pre-exist.

type C virogenes code for the production of particles secreted by the cell and contain specific viral proteins, a reverse transcriptase, and a high molecular weight RNA, their study appears to offer unique possibilities for purifying a discrete set of cellular genes and their products.

II. ISOLATION OF ENDOGENOUS PRIMATE TYPE C VIRUSES

Six separate isolates of infectious baboon type C virus have been obtained by cocultivation of kidney, lung, testes, and placenta from several different species of baboon (*Papio hamadyas* and *Papio cynocephalus*) using suitable permissive host cell lines. These isolates are all morphologically and biochemically typical of mammalian type C viruses, but are distinctly different by immunologic and nucleic acid hybridization techniques from all other previously studied type C viruses (*4, 16*). Furthermore, the six isolates are all highly related to each other by host range, viral neutralization, and interference, and by immunologic and nucleic acid hybridization criteria. [³H]DNA transcripts prepared from three of the baboon type C virus isolates hybridize completely to DNA extracted from various tissues of several different healthy baboons. These data suggest that these type C virus isolates are, indeed, endogenous viruses of baboons.

If the baboon type C viruses were truly endogenous primate viruses and had evolved, then it appears reasonable to suspect that other Old World monkeys that are close relatives to the baboon would have related virogene sequences in their DNA. Those primate species less related to baboons taxonomically would be expected to have much more extensive mismatching of their virogene sequences. The prosimians evolved from primitive mammalian stock roughly 60–80 million years ago. The New World monkey branch diverged from the common stem leading to both the apes and the Old World monkeys approximately 50 million years ago. The Old World monkeys (which include the baboon species) have been separated from the great apes and from man for 30–40 million years.

Hybridization studies employing an endogenous baboon type C viral [³H]DNA probe were used to detect type C viral nucleic acid sequences in primate cellular DNA. Sequences related to those of the baboon type C virus are found in all other Old World monkey species, higher apes, and, of particular importance, they are also found in man. The results presented support the conclusion that, within the primates, type C viral genes have evolved as the species have evolved, with virogenes from more closely related genera and families showing more sequence homology than those from distantly related taxons. The ubiquitous presence of endogenous type C virogenes among anthropoid primates and their evolutionary preservation for at least 30–40 million years suggest that such genes provide functions with a selective advantage to the species possessing them. They clearly have evolved in primates over the past 30–40 million years as stable cellular elements (5).

III. TRANSMISSION OF TYPE C GENES
BETWEEN DISTANTLY RELATED SPECIES

The endogenous type C viruses of baboons and domestic cats are related, but can be distinguished by biologic and immunologic criteria and by partial nucleic acid sequence homology. Virogene sequences in the DNA of Old World monkeys and domestic cats also show a degree of relatedness not shared by the unique sequence DNA of these species. Genes related to the nucleic acid of an endogenous domestic cat type C virus (RD-114) are found in the cellular DNA of anthropoid primates while many members of the cat family Felidae lack these sequences (Table 5). Endogenous viruses from

Table 5. Relationship between cat and baboon endogenous type C virus

1. The cat (RD-114/CCC) and baboon virus groups are *related but distinct* from one another by:
    a. viral DNA-RNA hybridization,
    b. inhibition of polymerase activity by antibody,
    c. antigencity of the p30 protein,
    d. viral interference,
    e. viral neutralization.
2. Cat and baboon unique sequence DNA markedly different, species diverged from one another over 80 million years ago.
3. Cat (RD-114/CCC) virus DNA transcripts hybridize to the DNAs of *all* Old World monkeys and apes, and to the DNAs of domestic cats and certain other felis species.
4. Baboon (M/M28) virus DNA transcripts hybridize to the DNAs of all Old World monkeys, higher apes, and man, and to DNAs of those felis species that contain RD-114 related sequences.

one group of mammals (primates) are thus concluded to have infected and become part of the germ line of an evolutionarily distant group of animals, ancestors of the domestic cat (6). The data demonstrate that viral genes from one group of animals can give rise to infectious particles that not only can integrate into the DNA of animals of another species, but can also be incorporated into the germ line (germ line inheritence of acquired virus genes). If viral gene sequences can be acquired in this way it is possible that type C viruses have served to introduce other genes from one species to another, and may provide an important mechanism by which species acquire new genetic information.

IV.   DETECTION OF ENDOGENOUS TYPE C
VIRAL GENE PRODUCTS IN PRIMATES INCLUDING MAN

Competitive radioimmunoassays that detect the major viral structural protein (p30) of baboon type C viruses also detect viral antigen in certain normal baboon tissues, in a normal stumptail macaque spleen, and a rhesus ovarian carcinoma. The p30 antigen from these tissues is closely related by several immunologic criteria to the p30 protein of baboon type C viruses. The results indicate that normal primate tissues translate at least one viral structural protein (9).

Partially purified extracts from 33 human tumors of several histologic types were used as competing antigens in a radioimmunoassay for the p30 protein of endogenous baboon type C virus. Antigens immunologically related to the p30 protein of the M7 baboon virus were detected in two tumors (a lymphoid lymphoma and an ovarian carcinoma). Like viral p30 antigens previously identified in tissues of several other primates, the antigens found in human tumors cross-react with the p30 protein of the RD-114 virus but are unrelated by similar immunologic criteria to the p30 proteins of several other mammalian type C viruses. Gel filtration shows that most of the antigenic activity cochromatographs with authentic p30 protein. These results, along with those showing nucleic acid sequences related to those of an endogenous primate type C virus in the DNA of human cells, make it clear that humans, like other primates, have type C viral sequences in their genomes and can, in some circumstances, express at least one type C viral protein (10).

V. THE POSSIBLE ROLE OF VIRUSES AS
NATURAL TRANSMITTORS OF GENES BETWEEN SPECIES

In recent months considerable interest has been focused on the possibilities and risks associated with the introduction of new genes into the germ line of a species. Genes can be inserted into or deleted from bacterial viruses in the laboratory by simple chemical manipulation. But what is known about the natural role of viruses as transmittors of genes in higher organisms?

In our laboratory in the past year we have developed evidence, as described above, that shows that RNA tumor virus (type C virus) genes have been maintained as stable endogenous genetic elements in primates, including man, for at least 30–40 million years. Viruses from an ancestor of the modern Old World monkeys also could be shown to have entered the germ line of ancestors of the domestic cat (Table 6). From the relatives of the domestic cat that have this virus and from those that did not acquire it, we have concluded that the infection occurred 3–10 million years ago somewhere in Africa or in the Mediterranean Basin region. Because of the stability of the viral gene sequences when they are incorporated into cellular DNA, events that have occurred millions of years ago still can be recognized by examining the genetic information of the virus and that of the host cell.

More recently, our laboratory has found a second example of gene transmission between species, in this case from an ancestor of the mouse to an ancestor of the domestic pig. Pig cell cultures produce type C viruses that can be shown to be genetically transmitted

Table 6. Examples of transmission of type C virus genes between species

Donor	Recipient	Genetically transmitted in recipient
Primate (Old World monkey)	Felis (ancestor of the domestic cat)	Yes
Rodent (mouse ancestor)	Pig ancestor	Yes
Rodent (asian Mouse M. caroli)	Primates and humans	No

and present in all pig tissues in multiple copies in the cellular DNA. Close relatives, such as the European wild boar and the African bush pig, have closely related viral genes in their DNA. It can be shown that this virus was acquired by an ancestor of the pig from a small rodent related to the mouse.

The genetically transmitted type C virus of the Asian mouse species, *Mus caroli,* can be shown to be closely related to the cancer-producing infectious primate type C viruses from gibbons, woolly monkeys, and, perhaps, humans (8).

That viruses can transmit themselves between the DNA of very different species has been established as a result of experiments in our own laboratory in the past year. That they can carry cellular gene sequences from cell to cell also has been clearly demonstrated. That this transmission of cellular gene information *between species* has been a major force in evolution remains a speculation without, at the moment, any direct proof.

Viruses are unique in that they can serve to carry information between genetically isolated species. Classic Darwinian evolution deals with changes that occur by mutation and selection, duplication, and rearrangement; the genetic information of a species can be changed and rearranged, but not added to from the outside. Viruses, such as the RNA tumor viruses, offer the possibility of additions of new gene sequences to a species. The type C viruses, as a group, are uniquely suited for this role since they must incorporate into the cellular DNA in order to replicate and they also do not kill the

Table 7. Possible functions of genetically transmitted virogenes in normal cells

1. Activation of oncogenic information, while inappropriate in adult tissue, plays a normal role during differentiation and development.

2. The integrated virus serves to protect the species against related, more virulent infectious type C viruses.

3. Virus activation, being linked to transformation, protects the animal by altering the cell membrane. The released virus could alert the immune system making the transformed cells more susceptible to immunologic control.

4. As conveyors of genetic information between species they may have had an evolutionary role. Only this group of viruses has been shown to transmit genes between germ cells of different species under natural conditions.

cells they infect. Each time they move from cell to cell they have the possibility of carrying with them host cell genes. They provide a means of communication between cells of different species and different phyla and they serve to keep a species in communication with its ecologic neighbors as well as genetic neighbors. Some of the possible normal functions that the virogene system may be involved in are summarized in Table 7.

Of course these same genes can transmit information that may disrupt normal cellular control and, by so doing, lead to the development of cancer in the individual. The cases of genetic significance, however, are when the new genes are incorporated into the germ line. The ease with which type C viruses can pick up host genes and can cross species barriers along with the general lack of lethal effect of these viruses makes them ideally suited for this kind of role.

Laboratory-created viruses might facilitate the incorporation of genes of particular interest, but clearly viruses have had that capability long before the arrival of molecular biologists, in fact, long before modern man appeared on the earth. Mammalian germ cells, then, our experiments show, are susceptible to viral-mediated acquisition of new genetic information.

LITERATURE CITED

1. Aaronson, S. and G. J. Todaro (1968). Science 162:1024–1026.
2. Aaronson, S., J. Hartley, and G. J. Todaro (1969). Proc. Nat. Acad. Sci. U.S.A. 64:87–94.
3. Baltimore, D. (1970). Nature 226:1209–1211.
4. Benveniste, R. E., M. M. Lieber, D. M. Livingston, C. J. Sherr, G. J. Todaro, and S. S. Kalter (1974). Nature 248:17–20.
5. Benveniste, R. E. and G. J. Todaro (1974). Proc. Nat. Acad. Sci. U.S.A. 71:4513–4518.
6. Benveniste, R. E. and G. J. Todaro (1974). Nature 252:456–459.
7. Huebner, R. and G. J. Todaro (1969). Proc. Nat. Acad. Sci. U.S.A. 64:1087–1094.
8. Lieber, M. M., C. J. Sherr, G. J. Todaro, R. E. Benvensite, R. Callahan, and H. G. Coon (1975). Proc. Nat. Acad. Sci. U.S.A., in press.
9. Sherr, C. J., R. E. Benveniste, G. J. Todaro (1974). Proc. Nat. Acad. Sci. U.S.A. 71:3721–3725.
10. Sherr, C. J. and G. J. Todaro (1974). Proc. Nat. Acad. Sci. U.S.A. 71:4703–4707.
11. Temin, H. M. and S. Mizutani (1970). Nature 226:1211–1213.
12. Temin, H. M. (1971). Ann. Rev. Microbiol. 25:609–648.

CHAPTER 3

Viruses and Breast Cancer

D. H. Moore

The existence in human milk and in human breast tumors of viruses with properties similar to those of the murine mammary tumor viruses (MuMTV) seems no longer to be questionable. This finding is quite separate, however, from the as yet unproved hypothesis that these viruses are etiologic agents in human breast cancer.

I. MURINE MAMMARY TUMOR VIRUSES

A. Biological Differences in MuMTVs

It is now evident that MuMTV represents a family of closely related viruses. The infectivity of MuMTV in a particular mouse strain depends on the source of the virus, and, conversely, the receptivity to a particular MuMTV varies greatly with the mouse strain (Tables 1 and 2).

Endogenous viruses found in high-mammary-tumor strains such as A, C3H, and RIII, demonstrable after the milk-transmitted virus is removed by foster nursing, were thought to be noninfectious (*16, 28, 29, 31*). It is now evident, however, that older mice of these substrains (Af, C3Hf, and RIIIf), after they have had several litters, secrete large quantities of virus in their milk. Although these viruses are noninfectious in the strains in which they are endogenous, they are highly infectious in mice of certain other strains (Table 2).

As shown by Tables 1 and 4 (below), BALB/c and RIIIf mice are resistant to intraperitoneal inoculations of the virus of RIII milk

This research was supported by Contract NO1-CP-33339 and Grant CA-08740 from the National Cancer Institute, General Research Support Grant FR-5582 from the Division of Research Facilities and Resources, and Grant-In-Aid M-43 from the State of New Jersey.

45

Table 1. Infectivity[a] titrations of RIII and BALB/cfC3H skim milk[b] in different mouse strains

Recipient strain	No. of mice infected/no. mice at risk (%)		
	10^{-1}	10^{-2}	10^{-3}
RIII			
C57BL	11/23(48)	13/26(50)	20/27(74)
BALB/c	2/15(13)	2/17(12)	10/31(33)
RIIIf	0/20(0)	0/18(0)	2/27(8)
Af	16/20(80)	18/19(95)	20/20(100)
BALB/cfC3H			
C57BL	3/18(17)	1/15(7)	0/15(0)
BALB/c		12/14(86)	12/15(80)
Af	11/14(79)	15/15(100)	13/17(76)
RIIIf	4/18(22)	5/15(33)	11/18(61)

[a]Infectivity determined by immunodiffusion test of MuMTV antigen in the milk of the inoculated mice taken after the 3rd litter (8).

[b]Skim milk diluted with phosphate buffered NaCl solution containing 0.1% bovine serum albumin. Test mice (3–5 weeks old) inoculated with 0.1 ml intraperitoneally.

Table 2. Infectivity[a] titrations of Af, RIIIf, and Af + RIIIf mixed (8th–10th lactation) skim milk in three different mouse strains

Recipient strain	No. mice infected/no. mice at risk			
	Control (PBS)	10^{-1}	10^{-2}	10^{-3}
Af				
C57BL	0/14(0)	1/17(6)	1/15(7)	0/18(0)
BALB/c	0/19(0)	5/18(28)	3/16(19)	0/18(0)
RIIIf	2/20(10)	7/20(35)	15/17(88)	12/18(67)
RIIIf				
C57BL	0/16(0)	2/14(14)	0/15(0)	1/17(6)
BALB/c	0/19(0)	19/20(95)	18/20(90)	20/20(100)
Af	2/19(11)	14/14(100)	17/17(100)	17/17(100)
Af + RIIIf				
C57BL	0/17(0)	1/12(8)	0/17(0)	0/17(0)
BALB/c	0/17(0)	18/18(100)	11/19(58)	3/16(19)

[a]See footnotes in Table 1.

Table 3. Infectivity[a] titration of ninth lactation RIIIf milk in C57BL mice

Dilutions No. infected/no. tested (%)					
10^{-2}	10^{-3}	10^{-4}	10^{-5}	10^{-6}	10^{-7}
1/20(5)	0/20(0)	2/18(11)	1/18(6)	2/19(10)	1/19(5)

[a]See footnotes in Table 1.

whereas C57BL mice are susceptible (24). The host spectrum of susceptibility for C3H virus carried in BALB/c (BALB/cfC3H) is very different from that of RIII. It is not known why the RIIIf mice (Table 1) are resistant to inoculations with the virus (RIII) that was secreted in their milk so abundantly until the substrain (RIIIf) was started by foster-nursing a litter of newborns on a C57BL mother. If, however, a litter of newborn RIIIf mice is foster-nursed on RIII mothers, they and their progeny are all infected, i.e., the high tumor line is restored. Unlike RIII milk, RIIIf milk is not infectious by the intraperitoneal route in C57BL mice but is very infectious in the BALB/c and Af lines (Tables 2 and 3).

Newborn C57BL females were substituted for the males of newborn litters delivered by older (6th–11th litter; milk contained virions and viral antigen) RIIIf mothers, so that they were nursing both their own daughters along with the C57BL. Of the 46 foster-nursed C57BL females that were bred to C57BL males, none expressed MuMTV antigen in the 3rd or 6th lactation milks nor did any develop tumors. Of the 67 RIIIf females (bred to RIIIf males), 8 (12%) expressed MuMTV antigen (4 were littermates) at the 3rd lactation and 12 (18%) at the 6th lactation. Unlike the infectivity of RIII virus, the infectivity of RIIIf virus was not affected by route of inoculation.

In another experiment the effect of extended dilutions on the infectivity of RIIIf milk in C57BL mice was tested. The milk used was taken at the 9th lactation and was shown to be positive for viral antigen by the immunodiffusion test. The results are shown in Table 3. For comparison the infectivity of RIII standard virus in C57BL mice is shown in Table 4.

B. Infectivity of Tissue Culture Fluids

When tissues from mouse mammary tumors are adapted to tissue culture they produce virions in quantities depending on several

Table 4. Infectivity[a] titration of purified[b] RIII virus in C57BL mice

	No. infected/no. at risk (%)					
10^{-1}	10^{-2}	10^{-3}	10^{-4}	10^{-5}	10^{-6}	10^{-7}
14/19(74)	14/18(78)	20/20(100)	15/18(83)	9/18(50)	4/18(22)	1/15(7)

[a] See footnotes in Table 1.
[b] Sucrose density gradient purified.

Table 5. Titrations[a] of supernatant fluid from cultures of BALB/cfC3H cells in BALB/c and C57BL mice

Hydrocortisone ($10\ \mu g/ml$)	No. infected/no. at risk (%)					
	10^{-3}	10^{-4}	10^{-5}	10^{-6}	10^{-7}	10^{-8}
			BALB/c			
Without	7/15(47)	7/16(44)	5/14(36)	4/14(29)	4/16(29)	0/15(0)
With	7/15(47)	2/15(13)	4/16(25)	3/15(20)	5/15(33)	4/16(25)
			C57BL			
Without	0/15(0)	1/17(6)	0/15(0)	0/12(0)	1/18(6)	0/15(0)

[a] See Table 1.

factors including the mouse strain from which they are derived (*19–21*). The milk from RIII mice contains about 10^{12} virions per milliliter and is the best source of virions, but RIII cells in vitro are a relatively poor source when compared with cells from BALB/cfC3H tumors. The concentration of virions in culture fluid can be enhanced by the addition of hydrocortisone and dexamethasone (*15*), but the infectivity of culture fluids is dependent on the mouse strain used for assay and does not seem to be very well correlated with virion concentration, as is illustrated in Table 5. When tested in BALB/c mice the culture-produced virus does not infect as does the milk transmitted virus of BALB/cFC3H (see Table 1) because none of the dilutions give an incidence of more than 50%, although some infectivity extends to dilutions of 10^{-7} or 10^{-8}. Particle counts on the fluids were estimated at 4.7×10^9 and 1.5×10^9 virions per milliliter with and without hydrocortisone, respectively. In C57BL mice, BALB/cf C3H fluid is essentially noninfectious.

C. MuMTV (From RIII Milk) Infection of Cells in Vitro

In vitro cultured cells can be infected with RIII mammary tumor virus. Recently an established line of cat kidney cells (CRFK-F2) (*10*) was infected (*18*). The cells were epithelial and doubled their population in 48 hr when placed in Hanks Eagle's medium supplemented with 10% fetal calf serum and 10 μg of insulin per milliliter. The inoculum was Ficoll density-gradient-purified virus from RIII milk. Virus was diluted to 10^{-2} in Hanks Eagle's medium containing 5 μg tetracycline per milliliter. No morphologic differences were observed between the infected and control cell lines. They grew at the same rate and were passaged once a week. MuMTV antigen was detected by immunofluorescence test of supernatant fluid 1 after inoculation, and typical B-particles were found budding from the cell membrane. Fluorescein labeled anti-MuMTV rabbit globulin showed that a specific MuMTV antigen existed on the surface of 10% of the cells, and this ratio rose to 25% after 3 months of cultivation. The infected cell lines have continued to produce virus for almost 2 years. Mammary tumors have developed in mice inoculated with the supernatant fluid. The addition of hydrocortisone (10 μg/ml) to the culture fluid increased virus 8-fold. That the cells were indeed cat cells was substantiated by chromosome counts (36–38 chromosomes). Anti-mouse cell serum tested on normal and infected CRFK-F2 cells had no significant cytotoxic effect. The isoenzyme pattern from these cells was found to be different from that of mouse, rat, hamster, and human cells. The infection of CRFK-F2 cells with MuMTV has been repeated.

D.   Possible Contagion of MuMTV in Susceptible Mice

In order to investigate the contagiousness of MuMTV, 3–5-week-old C57BL mice were maintained in the same boxes with retired, non-lactating RIII breeders. After 5 weeks the C57BL mice were sepa-rated from the MuMTV-bearing RIII females and normally bred with C57BL males. Two of 36 C57BL females were infected, as indicated by MuMTV antigen in the 3rd and also in the 6th lactation milks. In a similar experiment where young BALB/c mice lived with retired BALB/cfC3H breeders, 2 of 36 demonstrated viral antigen in both 3rd and 6th lactation milks. Normally neither C57BL nor BALB/c mice have ever shown viral antigen in their milks. The results thus far support previous evidence for horizontal transmission of MuMTV (4).

E.   Immunization of Mice with Inactivated MuMTV

Laboratory mice may be divided into three classes: (1) those that receive infectious virus through their mother's milk and have a high

Table 6. Effect of a single intramuscular vaccination[a] of RIIIf and Af mice

	No. mice positive/total no. mice (%)		
	MTV antigen in milk at 6th lactation	Tumors	
		at age 16 mo	at age 18 mo
RIIIf controls	40/150(27)	11/135(8.1)	16/124(12.9)
RIIIf vaccinated	10/171(5.9)	3/142(2.1)	7/134(5.2)
Effectiveness of vaccine	78%	74%	60%
Af controls	37/183(20)	11/168(6.6)	19/152(12.5)
Af vaccinated	11/180(6.1)	3/181(1.7)	8/170(4.7)
Effectiveness of vaccine[b]	70%	74%	62%

[a]Vaccines 67B and 67C were used in these experiments.

[b] $\dfrac{\%\ \text{infected (controls)} - \%\ \text{infected (vaccinees)}}{\%\ \text{infected (controls)}}$

incidence of mammary tumors relatively early in life, (2) those that do not receive infectious virus in their mother's milk but have an intermediate incidence of mammary tumors apparently as a result of the expression of the MTV genome carried in all mice, and (3) those that neither express virus nor develop tumors. Mice that receive large quantities of virus in their mother's milk from the time of birth are apparently tolerant to the viral antigens and are not immunized by vaccination (7). The other two classes, however, can be immunized (7). In a recent experiment, 400 weanling RIIIf females were divided into two groups of mixed littermates. One-half of the mice were immunized with 14 μg of purified formalin inactivated MTV from RIII milk, mixed with Freund's complete adjuvant (in other experiments, 1 μg of vaccine was found to be effective). Similarly, 400 Af mice were divided into two groups, one group being immunized and the other kept as controls. Table 6 and Figure 1 show the difference in the viral expression in milk

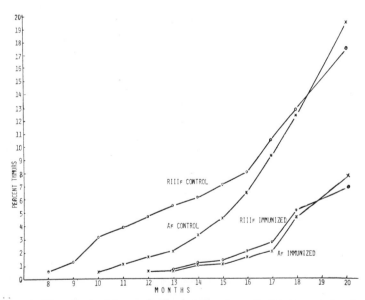

Figure 1. The effect of immunization on the percent of tumors appearing as a function of age (months) in two mouse strains carrying gamete transmitted (endogenous) MuMTV. Female mice (200) of each strain were vaccinated intramuscularly with 14 μg of formalin inactivated MuMTV in Freund's complete adjuvant at age 1 month. 200 littermates of each strain were maintained as controls. All were normally bred.

and the tumor incidence in two substrains that have a low incidence of mammary tumors.

An example of immunization of group 3 mice is shown in Table 7. Immunization before challenge with active virus completely protects these mice.

II. HUMAN MAMMARY TUMOR VIRUS

Whether there is a similar family of related viruses associated with human breast cancer, or whether they are involved in the etiology of malignancies of the human breast, or whether they can be blocked by immunization are questions as yet unanswered. Nevertheless, there are several pieces of evidence for the existence in human milk and breast tumors of viruses with properties similar to MuMTV. Since this evidence recently has been reviewed (12, 23), they will be mentioned here only briefly, with emphasis on the most recent unpublished data.

Although there have been conflicting reports concerning the presence of MuMTV-like particles in human materials (5, 9, 13, 32, 34), the first strong evidence that such a virus existed came from

Table 7. MTV specificity of protective (immunizing) antigen: Immunization with MTV-Vac$_1$[a] versus MTV-free mouse milk

Immunization (4–8 wk)	Challenge (8–10 wk)	Infective incidence[b]	
		Mice infected / Mice tested	Percent infected
PBS + FCA[c]; 0.2 ml	RIII MTV; 0.1 ml[d]	13/16	81
C57BL milk + FCA; 0.2 ml	RIII MTV; 0.1 ml	14/18	78
RIII milk + FCA; 0.2 ml	RIII MTV; 0.1 ml	16/19	84
RIIIf/C57BL milk + FCA; 0.2 ml	RIII MTV; 0.1 ml	14/14	100
Vac$_1$ + FCA; 0.1 ml	RIII MTV; 0.1 ml	0/42	0

[a]Formalin-inactivated, purified RIII MTV

[b]Detection of MTV antigen in milk of test mice at 3rd lactation (immunodiffusion assay)

[c]Freund's complete adjuvant

[d]Skim milk diluted $10^{-3.5}$

morphologic studies (*13, 25*). The number of virions (type B particles) liberated in human milk is extremely small. Mouse milk from high-mammary-tumor strains such as RIII contain about 10^{12} virions per milliliter. Human milk, on the contrary, contains less than 10^6 particle, which is below the limit of detectability by most procedures used in electron microscopy. Thin sections of pellets of purified particles show more virus-like particles than negatively stained dispersions. In section, it is often difficult to distinguish between B particles, C particles, and cytoplasmic debris. In negative stain, however, the 10-nm knobbed projections, which cover the outer viral membrane at a spacing of about 7.2 nm, make identification of uninjured virions unmistakable. Examination of milk specimens from more than a thousand women have revealed only 16 of these unquestionable structures. Explanations for these disparate observations among the different workers and for the paucity of B particles include the fact that humans do not produce the quantity of virus that mice do and the finding that most human milks contain virulytic factors that are very destructive to the morphologic integrity, biological activity, and the RNA-directed DNA polymerase (RDDP) activity of MuMTV and other viruses when added to these milks (*14, 33*). Human milks destroy not only MuMTV but other viruses such as Japanese B-encephalitis and Friend and Rauscher leukemia viruses (*14*), and it is likely that they destroy any human RNA virus in the same way.

A. RNA-Directed DNA Polymerase (RDDP)

This polymerase, a characteristic of RNA tumor viruses, has been found in human milk by many investigators (*11, 22, 36, 37*). The RDDP found in human milk particles varies greatly from one milk specimen to another, and it has been found that milk stored in the breast (fore milk) contains much less RDDP than the milk taken by continued aspiration (hind milk). This indicates that viral deterioration takes place within the breast (*22*).

The use of a synthetic template poly(rC)·oligo(dG) has been found to be more sensitive and also more specific for the RDDPs. This template has also provided a means of distinguishing between the enzyme of mammalian type C particles and that associated with the MuMTV particle by their preference for one of the two cations, Mg^{++} or Mn^{++}, for activity. The differences in poly(rC)·oligo(dG) directed [^{3}H]dGTP incorporation in the presence of the two different cations have been investigated by Dion et al. (*11*) and their results are reproduced in Table 8.

Sarkar found that it was possible to separate a mixture of B particles (MuMTV) from C particles (Rauscher leukemia virus) because of a difference in the buoyant densities of most of the particles of each type (*35*). The optical density of fractions recovered from a CsCl gradient after a mixture was centrifuged, is reproduced in Figure 2. Electron microscopic examination of the fractions showed that most of the B particles were in the density range of 1.18–1.22 and the C particles were at lower densities. In a similar fraction of particles from a pool of human milk, Dion et al. (*11*) found that Mg^{++} activated RDDP was associated with

Table 8. Cation preference for poly(rC) · oligo(dC) directed DNA synthesis

		Mg^{++a}	Mg^{++a}	Mg^{++}/Mn^{++b}
I.	Mammary tumor associated viruses			
	1. B-type viruses			
	RIII (mouse)[c]	29,100	2,274	12.8
	GR (mouse)	234,548	15,132	15.5
	A (mouse)	30,647	1,648	18.6
	C3H (mouse)	15,101	2,849	5.3
	2. B-C-type virus			
	MPMV (rhesus monkey)	8,493	401	21.2
	3. C-type viruses			
	R-35 (rat)	111	1,591	0.07
II.	Leukemia-sarcoma viruses			
	1. Mammalian C-type viruses			
	RLV (mouse)	8,802	49,042	0.18
	MSV (mouse)	922	10,102	0.10
	FLV (cat)	87,692	461,538	0.19
	GAL (gibbon ape)	2,317	5,312	0.44
	SSV (woolly monkey)	29,629	52,910	0.56
	2. Avian C-type viruses			
	AMV (chicken)	250,944	52,648	4.8
	RSV (chicken)	14,283	3,389	4.2

[a]Incorporation of [³H]dGTP (cpm) in the presence of optimal concentrations of Mg^{++} or Mn^{++}.

[b]Ratio of cpm of [³H]dGTP incorporation.

[c]Host is indicated in parentheses.

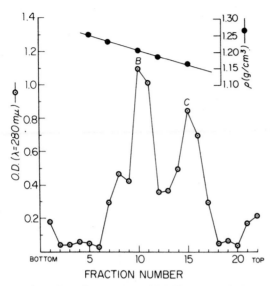

Figure 2. Separation of a mixture of B (MuMTV) and C (Rauscher leukemia virus) particles in a CsCl gradient. The particle types in each area were identified electron microscopically (from Ref. 35).

particles that banded at density 1.18–1.22 g/cm³ (Table 9). A correlation of RDDP activity with specific particles seen in the electron microscope would be helpful, but there is difficulty in doing this in light of the virulytic factors (*14, 33*) and nucleases (*22*) that occur in human milk. Attempts are being made to circumvent the action of these inhibitors.

B. Nucleic Acid Hybridization

Nucleic acid hybridization has proved to be a useful technique for the assay of genetic expression including tests for the relatedness of

Table 9. Cation preferences for pooled human milk fractions separated on CsCl gradients

	pmoles (^{3}H-dGMP) incorp./30 min		
Buoyant density in CsCl	Mg^{++} (8mM)	Mn^{++} (0.4mM)	Mg^{++}/Mn^{++}
1.16	0.04	0.23	0.17
1.18	0.36	0.07	5.11
1.22	0.34	0.18	1.88

viral genomes. The preparation of labeled DNA product complementary to endogenous viral RNA by the RDDP reaction constitutes a "probe" for the assay of nucleic acids from human tissues. Of 29 human breast tumor polysomal RNA preparations, 67% hybridized to a significant extent with labeled MuMTV DNA but not with Rauscher leukemia DNA probe (1). In contrast, no hybridization was detected between MuMTV DNA and polysomal RNAs derived from benign mastopathies, e.g., fibrocystic disease, fibroadenoma, gynaecomastia, or normal breast tissue. In addition, no RNA sequences complementary to MuMTV DNA have been found in human leukemias or sarcomas. These assays used isopycnic centrifugation in cesium sulphate gradients. In order to quantitate accurately the extent and fidelity of hybridization, Vaidya et al. (38) monitored total cellular RNAs of human mammary tumors and benign breast lesions by the stringent single-strand specific S1 nuclease technique. Of 17 breast cancer RNA preparations, 5 were found to protect more than 10% of the labeled MuMTV DNA probe against S1 nuclease-digested at $C_r t$ values (concentration of RNA in moles $\times$ time in seconds). The amount of MuMTV-related RNA found in some of the human tumors corresponded to 1.5–8 70 S equivalents per cell, which is similar to the number of MuMTV 70 S copies found in some of the mouse mammary tumors.

Presently, 36 human breast tissues have been monitored for MuMTV-related RNA and 11 had RNA that hybridized over 10% of the MuMTV probe. These fell into the following histopathologic classes: 3 of 6 (50%) were in situ, and 5 of 20 (25%) were invasive carcinomas, and 3 of 10 (30%) were nonmalignant breast lesions. In some cases two histopathologic types of tissue from the same breast were tested with the finding that the amount of MuMTV-related RNA could vary greatly. This indicates the importance of careful selection of tissues. There are preliminary suggestions of a correlation between well-differentiated appearance of tumor cells, family history of breast cancer, and the presence of MuMTV-related RNA. It may be concluded that these data do not constitute proof of a viral etiology for human breast cancer, but they provide strong evidence for the existence of virus-related information in human breast cancer. MuMTV is hormone dependent and is synthesized mainly in the breast tissue of mice, but the source of such a virus or related virus in human breast cancer is a major question. Unlike the mouse, it does not seem to be endogenous in man, because no virus-related DNA has as yet been found in human tissues. If it is not endogenous, it must be transferred either via mother's milk or by contagion. In light of its contagiousness in mice (see above), it may not be too early to consider contagiousness under favorable conditions of age and genetic susceptibility in humans.

C. Immunology

MuMTV related antigens in human materials have been indicated by several immunologic procedures. The first reported a neutralizing effect of human sera on MuMTV (6). In a preliminary study, sera from breast cancer patients showed a greater neutralizing effect than control sera, but later extensive tests indicated that about 25% of human sera had a neutralizing effect on MuMTV whether or not the sera came from breast cancer patients.

By indirect immunofluorescence it was observed that sera from 50% of breast cancer patients, 40% of relatives of some of those patients, and 15% of all donors reacted with mouse mammary cell cultures that were producing type B and C particles (30). It has been reported that sera from some women with breast cancer or with fibrocystic mastopathy caused slices of MuMTV-rich tumors to show an immunofluorescent reaction (26, 27). The human antibody seemed to be directed mainly against an antigen localized mainly in the intracytoplasmic A particles.

Similarity of antigens in the mouse virus and in human breast tissues is indicated by a leukocyte migration inhibition (LMI) test. This test is based on the premise that when lymphoid cells that have been previously sensitized to a specific antigen reencounter the same antigen, they respond by elaborating a factor that inhibits the in vitro movement of migrating cells. If the leukocyte fraction (buffy coat) from a cancer patient is placed in a small culture dish at a designated locus, the addition of the sensitizing antigen to the culture fluid causes a significant decrease in the measured area of migration compared with controls to which no antigen is added. This procedure has been used for comparing LMIs caused by cryostat sections of in situ and invasive human breast carcinomas with MuMTV (2, 3). Migration inhibition (> 25%) was found in 31% of the breast cancer patient's leukocytes tested against RIII virus-containing mouse milk in 33% of tests against homologous in situ breast cancer, in 29% of tests against autologous invasive breast cancer, and in 16% of tests against homologous invasive breast cancer tissues. MuMTV-free C57BL or RIIIf milks never caused leukocyte migration inhibition. It therefore appears that the antigenicity of human breast cancer tissue is due to a component that is antigenically similar to one associated with MuMTV. In direct support of this, Dion and Charney have prepared a MuMTV-related antigen from a large pool of many human milks. Highly concentrated samples of DEAE-cellulose fractions of detergent disrupted particles from human milk were tested against standard MuMTV antiserum (rabbit) by both micro-Ouchterlony and radioimmune assays. One of the fractions showed a strong line of identity with a MuMTV antigen by the Ouchterlony test and was identified in the radioimmune assay procedure as being MuMTV gp55-related (a glycoprotein of molecular weight 55,000). This is probably the strongest evidence for cross-reacting antigens in human and mouse particles and along with the extensive leukocyte migration inhibition data of Black et al. (2), the immunofluorescent data of Priori et al. (30) and Müller et al. (26), and the peroxidase-labeling data of Hoshino and Dmochowski (17), there seems to be little room for doubting the existence of cross-reacting MuMTV and human antigens. This is in agreement with the nucleic acid cross hybridizations and other evidences for MuMTV related virus in some human breasts.

LITERATURE CITED

1. Axel, R., J. Schlom, and S. Spiegelman (1972). Presence in human breast cancer of RNA homologous to mouse mammary tumour virus RNA. Nature 235:32–36.
2. Black, M. M., D. H. Moore, B. Shore, R. E. Zachrau, and H. P. Leis, Jr. (1974). Effect of murine milk samples and human breast tissues on human leukocyte migration indices. Cancer Res. 34:1054–1060.
3. Black, M. M., R. E. Zachrau, B. Shore, D. H. Moore, and H. P. Leis, Jr. (1975). Prognostically favorable immunogens of human breast cancer tissue: antigenic similarity to murine mammary tumor virus. Cancer 35:121–128.
4. Blair, P. B. and M. Lane (1974). Immunologic evidence for horizontal transmission of MTV. J. Immunology 113:1446–1449.
5. Calafat, J. and P. C. Hageman (1973). Remarks on virus-like particles in human breast cancer. Nature 242:260–262.
6. Charney, J. and D. H. Moore (1971). Neutralization of murine mammary tumour virus by sera of women with breast cancer. Nature 229:627–628.

7. Charney, J. and D. H. Moore (1972). Immunization studies with mammary tumor virus. J. Nat. Cancer Inst. 48:1125–1129.

8. Charney, J., B. D. Pullinger, and D. H. Moore (1969). Development of an infectivity assay for mouse mammary tumor virus. J. Nat. Cancer Inst. 43:1289–1296.

9. Chopra, H. C., P. Ebert, N. Woodside, J. Kvedar, S. Albert, and M. Brennan (1973). Electron microscopic detection of simian-type virus particles in human milk. Nature New Biol. 243:159–160.

10. Crandell, R. A., C. G. Fabricant, and W. A. Nelson-Rees (1973). Development, characterization and viral susceptibility of a feline (felis catus) renal cell line (CRFK). In Vitro 9:176–185.

11. Dion, A. S., A. B. Vaidya, and G. S. Fout (1974). Cation preferences for poly(rC) · oligo(dG)-directed DNA synthesis by RNA tumor viruses and human milk particulates. Cancer Res. 34:3509–3515.

12. Dmochowski, L. (1972). Viruses and breast cancer. Hosp. Prac. 7:73–81.

13. Feller, W. F. and H. C. Chopra (1971). Virus-like particles in human milk. Cancer 28:1425–1430.

14. Fieldsteel, A. H. (1974). Nonspecific antiviral substances in human milk active against arbovirus and murine leukemia virus. Cancer Res. 34:712–715.

15. Fine, D. L., J. K. Plowman, S. P. Kelley, L. O. Arthur, and E. A. Hillman (1974). Enhanced production of mouse mammary tumor virus in dexamethasone-treated 5-iododeoxyuridine-stimulated mammary tumor cell cultures. J. Nat. Cancer Inst. 52:1881–1886.

16. Heston, W. E. (1958). Mammary tumors in agent-free mice. Ann. N. Y. Acad. Sci. 931–942.

17. Hoshino, M. and L. Dmochowski (1973). Electron microscope study of antigens in cells of mouse mammary tumor cell lines by peroxidase-labeled antibodies in sera of mammary tumor-bearing mice and of patients with breast cancer. Cancer Res. 33:2551–2561.

18. Lasfargues, E. Y., B. Kramarsky, J. C. Lasfargues, and D. H. Moore (1974). Detection of mouse mammary tumor virus in cat kidney cells infected with purified B particles from RIII milk. J. Nat. Cancer Inst. 53:1831–1833.

19. Lasfargues, E. Y., B. Kramarsky, N. H. Sarkar, J. C. Lasfargues, and D. H. Moore (1972). An established RIII mouse mammary tumor cell line; kinetics of mammary tumor virus (MTV) production. Proc. Soc. Exp. Biol. Med. 139:242–247.

20. Lasfargues, E. Y., B. Kramarsky, N. H. Sarkar, J. C. Lasfargues, N. Pillsbury, and D. H. Moore (1970). Stimulation of mammary tumor virus production in a mouse mammary tumor cell line. Cancer Res. 30:1109–1117.

21. Lasfargues, E. Y., J. B. Sheffield, J. C. Lasfargues, and T. M. Daly (1973). Mammary tumor virus production in GR strain tumor cell cultures. J. Cell Biol. 59:187a.

22. McCormick, J. J., L. J. Larson, and M. A. Rich (1974). RNase inhibition of reverse transcriptase activity in human milk. Nature 251:737–740.
23. Moore, D. H. (1974). Evidence in favor of the existence of human breast cancer virus. Cancer Res. 34:2322–2329.
24. Moore, D. H., J. Charney, and J. A. Holben (1974). Titrations of various mouse mammary tumor viruses in different mouse strains. J. Nat. Cancer Inst. 52:1757–1761.
25. Moore, D. H., J. Charney, B. Kramarsky, E. Y. Lasfargues, N. H. Sarkar, M. J. Brennan, J. H. Burrows, S. M. Sirsat, J. C. Paymaster, and A. B. Vaidya (1971). Search for a human breast cancer virus. Nature 229:611–615.
26. Müller, M., C. Kemmer, S. Zotter, H. Grossmann, and B. Mitcheel (1973). Cross reaction between human breast cancer and mastopathy and murine mammary carcinoma: Localization of the antigens in type A particle virus. Arch. Geschwulstforsch. 41:100–106.
27. Müller, M., S. Zotter, H. Grossmann, and C. Kemmer. 1972. Antibodies in women with mammary carcinoma or proliferating mastopathy reacting specifically with an intracellular antigen of mammary tumour virus (MTV) producing tumours of mice. In: Colloque Recherches Fondamentales sur les tumeurs mammaires, J. Mouriquand, Ed., pp. 343–349. Institut National de la santé et de la recherche médicale, Paris.
28. Pitelka, D. R., H. A. Bern, S. Nandi, and K. B. DeOme (1964). On the significance of virus-like particles in mammary tissues of C3Hf mice. J. Nat. Cancer Inst. 33:867–885.
29. Pitelka, D. R., K. B. DeOme, and H. A. Bern (1960). Viruslike particles in precancerous hyperplastic mammary tissues of C3H and C3Hf mice. J. Nat. Cancer Inst. 25:753–777.
30. Priori, E. S., D. E. Anderson, W. C. Williams, and L. Dmochowski (1972). Immunological studies on human breast carcinoma and mouse mammary tumors. J. Nat. Cancer Inst. 48:1131–1135.
31. Pullinger, B. D. (1960). Tests for mammary tumour agent in C3Hf and RIIIf mouse strains. Br. J. Cancer 14:279–284.
32. Roy-Burman, P., R. W. Rongey, B. E. Henderson, and M. B Gardner (1973). Attempts to detect RNA tumour virus in human milk. Nature New Biol. 244:146.
33. Sarkar, N. H., J. Charney, A. S. Dion, and D. H. Moore (1973). Effect of human milk on the mouse mammary tumor virus. Cancer Res. 33:626–629.
34. Sarkar, N. H. and D. H. Moore (1972). On the possibility of a human breast cancer virus. Nature 236:103–106.
35. Sarkar, N. H. and D. H. Moore (1974). Separation of B and C type virions by centrifugation in gentle density gradients. J. Virol. 13:1143–1147.
36. Schlom, J., S. Spiegelman, and D. H. Moore (1971). RNA-dependent DNA polymerase activity in virus-like particles isolated from human milk. Nature 231:97–100.

37. Vaidya, A. B. (1973). Molecular biology of human milk. Science 180:776–779.
38. Vaidya,A. B., M. M. Black, A. S. Dion, and D. H. Moore (1974). Homology between human breast tumour RNA and mouse mammary tumour virus genome. Nature 249:565–567.

CHAPTER 4

734B: A Candidate
Human Breast Cancer Virus

C. M. McGrath, P. Furmanski,
J. Russo, J. J. McCormick, and M. A. Rich

I. INTRODUCTION

That RNA tumor viruses are in some way involved in neoplastic conversion of human breast epithelial cells has long been suspected. Until recently, the implication of a viral etiology in neoplastic breast disease was based largely on the numerous observations that RNA tumor viruses were etiologically involved in breast cancer of other animals. The demonstration that nucleotide sequences homologous to the virus known to cause cancer in mice are expressed in the messenger RNA fraction of malignant human breast cancers (5) strengthened the implication of virus gene expression as causal in human breast carcinogenesis.

The direct demonstration of viral etiology in human breast cancer has been frustrated by the inability to isolate endogenous RNA tumor viruses from breast cancer cells. An attempt to isolate such candidate human viruses and to evaluate their role in breast carcinogenesis is the subject of this chapter.

II. ISOLATION OF HUMAN BREAST CARCINOMA CELLS

At the outset of our studies we considered that the most favorable source of "endogenous" human breast cancer viruses would be

This work is being carried out with the support of Contract NOI-CP-33347 within the Virus Cancer Program of the National Cancer Institute, National Institute of Health, Public Health Service, and an institutional grant from the United Foundation of Detroit. The auhors acknowledge the cooperation of Dr. J. Gruber and the office of Program Resources and Logistics, National Cancer Institute.

human breast cancer cells and that the most favorable source of these cells would be a line of homogeneous breast cancer epithelium in continuous in vitro passage. Availability of such a line with a homogeneous breast carcinoma phenotype would allow both the standardization of techniques for virus recovery and yield the necessary amplification of gene expression. The use of cell lines derived from breast cancers necessitated the exercise of extreme care in establishing that the cultured cells were indeed human, mammary epithelial cells of neoplastic origin, free of adventitious viral contaminants.

The MCF-7 cell line was established from a pleural effusion of a patient with disseminated malignant adenocarcinoma of the breast (28). It has maintained its original polygonal epithelial growth characteristics through 160 serial passages. Ultrastructurally, the MCF-7 cell is classified as epithelial as evidenced by several markers including a well-developed junctional complex system between cells and epithelioid microvilli (3). The growth pattern and histoformative capacity of the cells in collagen-coated sponges resembles very closely that of the epithelial cells growing in the original pleural effusion and in the original adenocarcinoma (26).

MCF-7 cells have a human subtetraploid karyotype, exhibit human plasma membrane antigens, and synthesize the human, type B glucose-6-phosphate dehydrogenase isozyme (21, 28). The molecular weight of the 28 S ribosomal RNA of MCF-7 cells is identical to human ribosomal RNA and clearly distinguishable from that of mouse and other species (28).

MCF-7 cells possess specific 17 β-estradiol receptors (9). This activity is strongly suggestive of both a parenchymal endocrine origin, and a maintenance of that differentiative state throughout long-term cultivation in vitro. Recently, we detected α-lactalbumin synthesis in MCF-7 cells using an extremely specific and sensitive radioimmunoassay for the human milk protein (24). α-lactalbumin is the B protein in the lactose synthetase enzyme system and is a specific marker for differentiated mammary epithelial cells. Synthesis of this protein by MCF-7 cells is a strong indication that the MCF-7 cells are of breast epithelial derivation and have retained that differentiative phenotype in serial passage. It is conceivable that nonbreast cells could acquire such markers as a function of progressive dedifferentiation during serial cultivation. Such a hypothesis, however, is unlikely because it would require the ectopic synthesis of at least two markers for endocrine breast cell function within 40 passages of the cells in vitro.

The data germane to the human breast epithelial and neoplastic nature of MCF-7 are summarized in Table 1. Note that by several criteria the possibility of Hela cell contamination can be eliminated.

With the availability of homogeneous breast cancer epithelium as a substrate, we turned our attention to the isolation of human breast cancer viruses.

We have reported the isolation of an RNA tumor virus-like particle from supernatants of cultures of MCF-7 cells (20). Replication of the particle appeared to require a shift in incubation temperature. Whether the temperature shifts result in the induction of an endogenous viral genome directly from host DNA or the amplification of a low-level replicating virus is currently under study. The particles, banding with a buoyant density of 1.16–1.18 g/cm^3 in linear sucrose gradients, contain RNA with a molecular weight of $10–12 \times 10^6$, and a polymerase catalyzing the synthesis of DNA using high molecular weight RNA present in the particle as a template in the reaction. Immunofluorescence studies, using antisera to murine mammary tumor virus (MuMTV) structural antigens, revealed that an antigen immunologically indistinguishable from a MuMTV antigen was synthesized in MCF-7 carcinoma cells in association with the synthesis of the RNA tumor virus-like particle. The virus-like properties of the particle, called 734B, are more fully described below.

III. HOMOLOGY OF 734B WITH OTHER VIRUSES

A. Structure of 734B

We have identified particles in density-gradient bands of MCF-7 culture supernatants which resemble RNA tumor viruses (Figure 1, *a* and *b*). The particles, which band with a density of 1.17 ± 0.01 g/cm^3 are 100–110 nm in diameter with an electron-dense inner core, 65–90 nm in diameter. The core may be either centrically located as with C-type or immature B-type or ecentrically located as in the case of B-type particles (7). Spikes, as observed on MuMTV particles (7), or spines as described for human foamy viruses (1), have not been observed on these particles. The single factor that has precluded definitive association of these particles

Table 1. Characteristics of MCF-7 cells

Activity measured	Ref.	Reference cell	Indication
Membrane antigenicity	28	Balb/c lymphocytes(M)[a] Human lyphocytes(H)	Human
Karyotype and chromosomal markers	28, 21	D-562(H); HeLa(H) MCF-8(M)	Human; non-HeLa
Glucose-6-phosphate dehydrogenase	28	HeLa(H) MCF-8(M)	Human type B; non-HeLa
Molecular weight of ribosomal RNA	28	Primary human foreskin(H) MCF-8(M)	Human
Estrogen receptor	9	HeLa(H)	Endocrine, epithelial, non-HeLa
α-Lactalbumin synthesis	24	HeLa(H); Hep-2(H)	Human, mammary, ephithelial, non-HeLa
Growth in agar suspension	33	Normal mammary epithelial(H), (M) Malignant mammary epithelial(M)	Neoplastic
Concanavalin A mediated hemadsorption	33	Malignant mammary epithelial(M)	Neoplastic
Nucleus/cytoplasm size ratio	10	Malignant mammary epithelial(M), (H)	Neoplastic
Growth in sponge matrices	26	Original tumor; pleural effusion	Neoplastic, adenocarcinomatous

[a](M), mouse cell; (H), human cell.

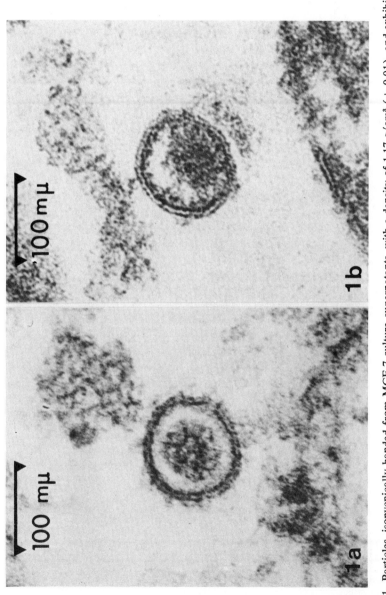

Figure 1. Particles, isopycnically banded from MCF-7 culture supernatants, with a density of 1.17 g/cm³ (± 0.01), and exhibiting RNA directed DNA polymerase (20) were prepared for transmission electron microscopy. The material was pelleted and fixed for 2 hr in glutaraldehyde-osmium tetroxideuranyl acetate, embedded in Epon and sectioned. × 250,000.

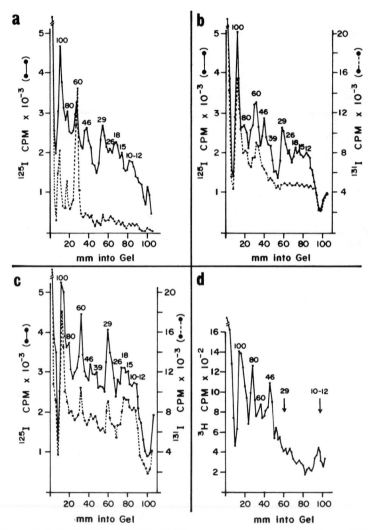

Figure 2. Polypeptides of 734B. 734B was isopycnically banded from MCF-7 culture supernatants as described (20). Material banding at densities between 1.13 and 1.15, 1.16–1.18, and 1.20–1.22 g/cm³ was collected and pelleted separately. These pellets were resuspended in 0.01 M Tris-HCl (pH 8.5) and divided into two aliquots. Assays for RNA and DNA directed DNA polymerases were performed on 20–40 µg of protein as described previously (20). The remainder of the material was disrupted in 0.5% Triton X-100, iodinated using chloramine T (14) and exhaustively dialyzed against Tris-HCl (0.01 M), NaCl (0.15 M), EDTA (0.001 M) buffer (pH 7.2). The samples were further solubilized in SDS in the presence of dithiothrestol (DTT) and urea and sized

with the RNA-dependent DNA polymerase activity of 734B (see below), has been their paucity in the gradient bands; to date, the small numbers of whole particles have made it impossible reproducibly to correlate reverse transcriptase activity with a particular morphologic entity.

We have recently completed an electrophoretic analysis of 734B polypeptides in polyacrylamide gels as a first step in protein isolation for antiserum production. The predominant polypeptides solubilized from 734B particles with Triton X-100 and ether are illustrated in Figure 2. Nine major polypeptides can be resolved in 10% acrylamide-sodium dodecyl sulfate (SDS) gels. These are proteins of 100,000, 80,000, 60,000, 46,000, 29,000, 26,000, 18,000, 15,000, and 10,000–12,000 molecular weight (Figure 2a). The p10–12[1] has not been resolved into component polypeptides in polyacrylamide gels, but p10 and p12 have been resolved by chromatography in Sepharose 6B columns equilibrated with 6 M guanidine-HCl (not shown). A polypeptide of 39,000 daltons has also occasionally been identifiable as separate from p46 (Figure 2c).

Four of the slowest migrating polypeptides as well as a component of p10–12 appear to be glycopeptides (Figure 2d). This was established by internally labeling 734B with glucosamine, solubilizing the labeled particles in detergent, and sizing the solubilized polypeptides in 10% SDS gels in a manner identical to that used for iodinated polypeptides (cf. Figure 2a).

The polypeptides described above were solubilized from particles with buoyant densities of 1.16–1.18 g/cm³ that contained 734B reverse transcriptase activity (RNA-dependent DNA poly-

---

[1]By convention (4), viral polypeptides are referred to by the prefix "p" (polypeptide) or "gp" (gylcopeptide) followed by the apparent molecular weight ($\times$ 10^{-3}).

---

in 10% SDS-polyacrylamide gels as described (15). In a, 1.16–1.18 g/cm³ particles (•——•) and particles pelleted from nonproducer MCF-7 culture supernatants (•–––•) are shown. In b, polypeptides of particles with a density of 1.16–1.18 g/cm³ (•——•) were co-electrophoresed with polypeptides of 1.20–1.22-g/cm³ particles (•–––•). In c, 1.16–1.18-g/cm³ particles (•——•) were co-electrophoresed with 1.13–1.15-g/cm³ particles (•–––•). In d, MCF⁺ cells were labeled with 20 µCi/ml D-[³H]-glucosamine (New England Nuclear, 12 Ci/mmol). Tritium-labeled particles with densities of 1.16–1.18 g/cm³ were solubilized in SDS as above and sized in 10% polyacrylamide gels.

merase, RDDP). To establish which of the polypeptides were viral and which were cellular, we compared these polypeptides with those found in similar gradient bands of material in which no RDDP activity could be demonstrated. High-speed pellets of supernatants from cloned non-734B producing MCF-7 sublines contained the three largest glycoproteins (Figure 2a, Table 2). Similarly, gradient bands with an average density of 1.20 g/cm^3 that exhibited no RDDP activity but were rich in cell fragments and exhibited DNA templated DNA polymerase activity (DDDP) also contained the three largest (slowest migrating) glycoproteins (Figure 2b). Noticeably absent from gel profiles of RDDP negative particles are the gp46, p39, p29, p26, p18, p15, and p10–12. Particles with densities of 1.13–1.15, which exhibited RDDP activity as well as DDDP activity, contained all nine major polypeptides associated with 1.16–1.18 particles (Figure 2c; Table 2). The association of the seven smaller polypeptides with 734B particles and their absence in homologous cell supernatants not producing 734B suggest their consideration as polypeptide markers for 734B. The specific origin of the larger glycoproteins is less clear at this time.

Table 2. Association of seven polypeptides with particles containing 734B RNA; dependent DNA polymerase[a]

Particle density	Resident polymerase	Solubilized polypeptides
1.13–1.15 g/cm^3	DDDP and RDDP	gp100, gp80, gp60, gp46, p39 p29, p26, p18, p15, p10, 12
1.16–1.18 g/cm^3	RDDP	gp100, gp80, gp60, gp46, p39 p29, p26, p18, p15, p10, 12
1.20–1.22 g/cm^3	DDDP	gp100, gp80, gp60
NP fluid pellet[b]	DDDP	gp100, gp80, gp60

[a]Particles of the designated densities were isopycnically banded in sucrose gradients, pelleted, and resuspended in 0.01 M Tris-HCl, pH 8.5. Assays for DNA-dependent DNA polymerases (DDDP) and RNA-dependent DNA polymerases (RDDP) were performed using 20–40 μg protein as described (20). RDDP activities were those heteropolymerization reactions insensitive to actinomycin D (100 μg/ml) and > 95% sensitive to pancreatic RNAase (cf. Table 6). DDDP reactions were those less than 30% RNAase sensitive and inhibited by actinomycin D (100 μg/ml). The remainder of the particles (about 10–50 μg of protein) recovered from sucrose gradients were solubilized, iodinated, and analyzed for constituent polypeptides as described in the legend for Figure 2.

[b]NP fluid pellet: pellet of 100,000 × g centrifugation of growth media from MCF-7 clone-1 that produces no 734B (20).

The polypeptides of 734B are remarkably similar in molecular weight to those of the Mason Pfizer monkey virus (MPMV) grown in human cells (Figure 3a). MPMV is an RNA tumor virus derived from a simian breast adenocarcinoma (2, 11) and is thought to be involved in malignant breast disease. MPMV is also found in some human tumor cell lines including Hela and Hep-2 (16, 17). To determine whether any or all of the 734B polypeptides were identical in molecular weight to either MPMV or MuMTV polypeptides, solubilized 734B polypeptides were co-electrophoresed with MPMV and MuMTV proteins in 10% SDS gels. As illustrated in Figure 3, the four major glycoproteins found in 734B preparations, including gp46, co-electrophoresed with corresponding MPMV polypeptides. The p26, a minor component of 734B, migrated with the major MPMV protein. Both particles contained p10–12 and a p18. Only the p15 of 734B is without a counterpart in MPMV. At least two polypeptides of 734B, the p15 and p10–12 coelectrophoresed with the corresponding polypeptides of MuMTV (Figure 3b). Despite the obvious similarities in molecular weights of several MPMV, MuMTV, and 734B polypeptides, differences do exist in the migration pattern of nonglycosylated polypeptides, especially the major nonglycosylated polypeptides of MuMTV (p28), MPMV (p26), and 734B (p29) (Figure 3, a–d), which makes identity between the three viruses unlikely.

B. Serologic Cross Reactions

Antisera prepared against two purified polypeptides of murine leukemia virus-Rauscher (MuLV) did not react with 734B-producing MCF-7 (MCF$^+$) cells in indirect immunofluorescence assays (Table 3). The two anti-MuLV p30 sera did, however, recognize interspecies leukemia virus determinants. Anti-gp69,71 likewise exhibited no reactivity for MCF$^+$ cells. The lack of reactivity with antisera against C-type internal (p30) and external (gp69, 71) virus polypeptides, suggests that 734B is not a C-type leukemia virus contaminant in MCF-7 cells.

Within either the leukemia or sarcoma C-type virus families, considerable interspecies homology appears to have been retained during host evolution. Murine type-C virus markers, for example, have been identified in simian viruses (6) and simian C-type markers and have also been identified in putative human viruses (12). The conservation of virion structural information in C-type viruses has

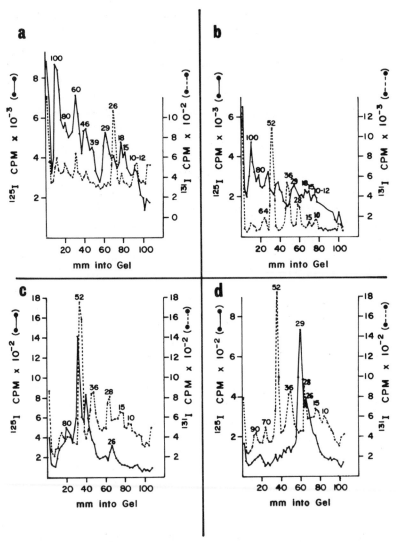

Figure 3. Co-electrophesis of 734B with MuMTV and MPMV polypeptides. All three viruses were obtained by isopycnic banding of tissue culture supernatants; MuMTV from Balb/cfc3H cultures; MPMV from NC37 cultures and 734B from MCF+ cells. Viruses were disrupted, iodinated, solubilized, and sized in 10% SDS-acrylamide gels as in Figure 2. In *a*, ^{125}I-labeled 734B (•———•) was co-electrophoresed with [181]I-MPMV (•----•); in *b*, [125]I-734B polypeptides (•———•) were co-electrophoresed with [181]I-MuMTV polypeptides

led to the construction of "affinity patterns" which suggest that human viruses belonging to a particular family of C-type viruses carry some murine C-type markers (*12*). Since mammary tumor viruses as cell-free entities have been isolated from relatively few host species, analyses of "viral affinity patterns" generated during progressive host evolution has not yet been possible for these viruses. Since the origin of MuMTV genes from host cell nucleic acids and the generation of diversity within the genome should be similar to that which occurs for endogenous C-type viruses, it is likely that "affinity patterns" exist within the B-type family of viruses and that some homology between human and nonhuman mammary tumor viruses might be observed. Efforts were therefore initiated to evaluate homology between 734B and nonhuman mammary cancer viruses. In addition to studies comparing 734B with MuMTV, a putative simian mammary tumor virus, the Mason Pfizer monkey virus (MPMV), was also studied. MPMV was isolated from a simian breast cancer (*2, 11*) and, as such, might be considered a relative to MuMTV. However, this virus, which is unrelated to C-type viruses (*12*), appears also to be unrelated to the murine mammary tumor virus (*2, 11*). At present its ancestry and biologic function remain uncertain.

To evaluate cross-reactivities with 734B, two MPMV antisera have been used in immunofluorescence assays. One was an unabsorbed antiserum prepared against detergent-disrupted MPMV grown in human (NC 37) cells. This serum reacted with MCF$^+$ cells. However, the antiserum reacted equally well in dilution experiments with any human cell tested including a cloned MCF$^-$ line, a foreskin fibroblast line, a throat adenocarcinoma line (Detroit 562), and uninfected NC37 cells, suggesting that the reaction was not entirely MPMV specific. An antiserum prepared against the major protein of MPMV (p26) did not react with MCF-7 cells at two 2-fold dilutions less than the terminal reactive dilution for NC37 cells infected with MPMV. Furthermore, extracts of MCF-7 cells have

---

(•----•); in *C,* partially purified ^{125}I-labeled gp60 and gp46 (which also contained some p26) were co-electrophoresed with ^{131}I-MuMTV polypeptides (•----•). In *d,* partially purified 734B p29 (•----•) (which also contained p26) was co-electrophoresed with MuMTV polypeptides (•----•). Partial purification of 734B polypeptides gp46 and p29 was effected by single-step chromotography of ^{125}I-734B polypeptides in sepharose 6B gel columns equilibrated with 6 M guanidine-HCl (*14*).

Table 3. Reactivity of MCF-7 cells with anti-viral antisera

Antiserum[a]	Reactivity (% cells fluorescent)					
	MCF-6[b]	Balb/cfc3H	NC37(MPMV)	MCF-7w	MCF-7cl-1	D562
MuLV p30-I	98–100	0	ND	0	ND	ND
MuLV p30-II	98–100	0	ND	0	ND	ND
MuLV gp69,71	98–100	0	ND	0	ND	ND
MPMV-TXX	0	0	100	75	75	98–100
MPMV p27	0	0	100	0	0	0
MuMTV-TXX(113A)	0	100	0	6	0	0
MuMTV-gp52	0	57	ND	0	0	ND
MuMTV-p27	0	72	ND	3–7	0	0
MuMTV-p27 Absorbed with MuMTV[c]	ND	1%	ND	0	ND	ND
MuMTV-p27 Absorbed with MuLV	ND	96	ND	3–5	ND	ND

[a]Description of antisera: Both anti-MuLV p30 sera were obtained through the Virus Cancer Program of the NIH (VCP) and both recognized interspecies determinants on p30; anti-MuLV gp69,71 was obtained from Dr. J. T. August; its reactivity for MuLV envelope antigens has been described (29); MPMV-TXX is an antiserum obtained through the SVCP and was prepared against detergent-disrupted MPMV grown in NC37 cells; anti-MPMV p27 was kindly provided by Dr. J. Yeh of Pfizer Labs; polyvalent anti-MuMTV (113A) has been described (20); anti-gp52 and anti-p27 of MuMTV were obtained through the SVCP; their reactivity against MuMTV has been described (22). With one exception each antiserum was used at two 2-fold dilutions less than that threshed dilution for reactivity against homologous virus-containing cells. Anti-MuMTV gp52 was used at a 1:4 dilution throughout.

[b]The cells used in these experiments have been described previously (20).

[c]Four absorptions with detergent disrupted MuMTV were required to reduce fluorescent to 1% levels in Balb/cfc3H cells.

not been active in competitive radioimmunoassays for MPMV p27. These data suggest that in spite of considerable similarity in molecular weight of polypeptides, 734B is immunologically distinct from MPMV.

To determine serologic cross-reactivity between 734B and MuMTV, one antiserum, prepared against detergent-solubilized MuMTV virions, was reacted with MCF$^+$ cells in immunofluorescence tests. This antiserum (113AV) contained antibodies reactive against determinants on the gp52, p28, p15, and p10–12 of MuMTV. This was determined by the electrophoresis in acrylamide-SDS gels of polypeptides that specifically bound to and eluted from sepharose 4B affinity column prepared with 113AV globulins. The results of the immunofluorescence tests are shown in Table 3. Determinants on one or all of the four MuMTV polypeptides recognized by 113AV appear to be synthesized by MCF-7 cells in association with 734B. The gp52 is the major surface polypeptide of MuMTV (22, 30), the p28 is the major internal polypeptide (22, 31), and the p15 appears, on the basis of its cosedimentation with MuMTV RNA and its high pI, to be the nucleoprotein of MuMTV. The p10–12 is a mixture of unresolved polypeptides of uncertain function in the virion.

The availability of antisera reactive against each of the two major MuMTV polypeptides (gp52 and p28) has expedited a more thorough analysis of cross-reactive 734B-MuMTV polypeptides. In immunofluorescence tests, anti-gp52 did not react with MCF$^+$ cells (Table 3). However, only 57% of MuMTV synthesizing Balb/cfc3H cells reacted with anti-gp52 at a 1:4 dilution, indicating a low (but specific) titer for that serum. Reactivity with anti-p28 was observed with MCF$^+$ cells. This reactivity was not observed with MuLV$^+$ Balb/c (MCF-6) cells at the dilution used, human nonbreast cells, nor MCF$^-$ (clone-1) cells. The reactivity for MCF$^+$ cells could be absorbed from anti-p28 serum with detergent-solubilized MuMTV. These results suggest that determinants cross-reactive with those of the major MuMTV core protein are present during 734B synthesis in MCF-7 cells.

To determine if the cross-reactive antigen synthesized in MCF$^+$ cells was an integral part of the 734B particle or only cell associated, radioimmunoassays were conducted using the p28 antiserum and cell-free 734B preparations.

Figure 4 illustrates the results of immunoprecipitation of 734B using anti-p28. Twenty-one percent of the total ^{125}I-734B polypeptides was precipitated at a serum dilution of 1:250; 50% precipitation occurred at a 1:750 dilution. Neither MPMV (not shown) nor MuLV polypeptides were precipitated under conditions in which the major internal polypeptides of those viruses were, respectively, 94% and 92% precipitable from the same preparations using homol-

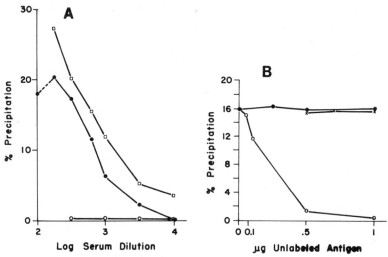

Figure 4. Immunoprecipitation of ^{125}I-734B by anti-MuMTV p28 sera. 734B was isopycnically banded from MCF-7 culture supernatants as described previously (20). Particles banding with a density of 1.17 ($\pm$ 0.01) g/cm^3, and exhibiting RDDP activity were disrupted in 0.5% triton and iodinated as described in the legend for Figure 2. Disrupted particles, exhibiting a polypeptide profile as in Figure 2a, were assayed for antigenic determinants recognizable by goat anti-p28 (22). Reactions were carried out by mixing 10,000 acid precipitable 734B cpm with anti-p28 in 0.01 M Tris-HCl (pH 7.2), 0.15 M NaCl, 100 μg/ml of bovine serum albumin (BSA). The secondary precipitation system was normal goat globulins and rabbit anti-goat IgG (Antibodies Incorporated, Davis, Calif.) at equivalence. All antigen–antibody reactions were for 1 hr followed by overnight refrigeration. The resulting pellets were collected by centrifugation and counted by gamma spectrometry. A, precipitation of ^{125}I-734B (• – – – •), ^{125}I-MuMTV (□ —— □), and ^{125}I-MuLV (Rauscher (○ —— ○) by anti-p28 as a function of anti-p28 concentration. The submaximal precipitation of ^{125}I-734B at a 1:100 serum dilution was due to a shift from equivalence to antigen (goat globulin) excess in the secondary system. B, competitive inhibition of 734B precipitation by disrupted MuMTV (○ —— ○), MPMV (• —— •), and MuLV (Rauscher, X —— X) as a function of competing antigen concentration. Competitions were saturation competitions executed by mixing anti-p28 with competing antigen for 1 hr before addition of ^{125}I-734B to the system.

ogous antisera. The precipitation of ^{125}I-734B was competitively inhibited with solubilized MuMTV polypeptides but not by MPMV or MuLV polypeptides (Figure 4B). These data suggest that determinants on the p28 of MuMTV are cross-reactive with determinants on polypeptides of the 734B particle.

Using a competitive radioimmunoassay composed of a primary ^{125}I-MuMTV–anti-p28 system we are evaluating the extent of cross-reactivity of p28 determinants for the two viruses. Preliminary data using 734B as competing antigen suggest that both the affinity of anti p28 for cross-reactive determinants and the number of determinants are different for the two viruses. This nonidentity would be consistent with the observation that the p28 of MuMTV does not coelectrophorese with the p29 of 734B, although considerable overlap in their size does exist (see Figure 3).

C. Nucleic Acid Sequence Relatedness

The appropriate design of molecular hybridization experiments depends to a large extent on whether one needs to illuminate absolute identity or merely similarity in the components to be compared. Most of our annealing studies to date have been directed toward determining if 734B was identical to particular nonhuman viruses. Our annealing conditions have, therefore, been stringent (high temperature, low salt). In these hybridization experiments, 734B-producing MCF-7 cells were used as the source of 734B RNA so as to provide sufficient material to carry the experiments to kinetic completion. When this RNA was reacted with certain DNA molecular probes (cDNA) prepared from MuMTV, hybridization occurred. The kinetics of association between one MuMTV cDNA and MCF$^+$ RNA is shown in Figure 5. The $C_r t_{1/2}$ of this association was $10^{3.2}$, nearly 10-fold greater than the $C_r t_{1/2}$ between this cDNA and Balb/cfc3H (MuMTV$^+$) tumor cell RNA. Maximum hybridization was 37% for MCF$^+$ RNA and 92% for Balb/cfc3H. Control cytoplasmic RNAs for annealing with MuMTV cDNAs were mouse 3T3 cell RNA and human placental RNA. Tables 4 and 5 summarize the results of hybridizations using several nonhuman, C-type, B-type, and MPMV, RNA tumor virus cDNAs. Three independently prepared mouse leukemia virus (MuLV-Rauscher) cDNAs failed to anneal more than 2% with MCF$^+$ RNA at a $C_r t$ of 10^4 (Table 4). This level of reaction should be considered nonspecific. The MPMV cDNA similarly failed to react with MCF$^+$ RNA (Table 4). Table

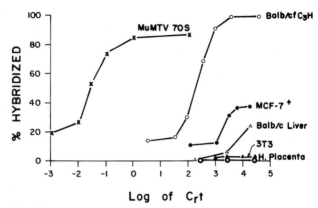

Log of $C_r t$

Figure 5. Hybridization of MuMTV cDNA B-19 to MCF-7 RNA. The MuMTV cDNA was prepared from isopycnically banded virus from RIII milk. Endogenous RNA directed DNA polymerase activity was obtained by addition of 0.25% Nonidet P40 to virions in the presence of 0.1 M Tris-HCl (pH 8.0), 10^{-4} M dCTP, dGTP, and dATP, 8×10^{-5} M [³H]TTP (New England Nuclear, 17–20 Ci/mol), 2×10^{-3} M MgCl₂, and 100 µg of actinomycin D (Merck) per ml. Reactions were for 1 hr at 37°C and were terminated with 0.5% SDS. DNA products were purified by pronase, RNAase, and NaOH treatments according to Ref. 32. RNA was prepared from MuMTV virions as described previously (19). RNA was prepared from cells by methods recommended in Ref. 32. These methods included pronase and DNAase treatment of RNA preparations. DNA-RNA hybridizations were conducted by mixing 500 cpm of cDNA with various concentrations of RNA in 0.25 M Tris-HCl (pH 7.4), 0.001 M EDTA, and 0.4 M NaCl. Reactions were at 68°C for 66 hr. $C_r t$ values were varied by changing RNA concentrations. Amount of hybridization was measured by S_1 digestion of unhybridized cDNA (32). $C_r t$ values were calculated as recommended in Ref. 8. Percent hybridizations shown are those with only scintillation counter backgrounds subtracted.

5 shows that not all MuMTV cDNAs have annealed with a single MCF⁺ RNA under stringent annealing conditions. The MuMTV cDNAs that did so, however, did not anneal with either 3T3 or human placental RNA. The T_m of the MuMTV cDNA-MCF⁺ hybrids formed in 0.4 M NaCl was 63° in 0.01 M Tris as compared with 66° for the homologous reaction (MuMTV cDNA-MuMTV RNA), indicating 2–3% mismatching in the MuMTV-MCF⁺ hybrid.

Having established that 734B is not identical to various known nonhuman RNA tumor viruses, we have begun to evaluate *similarities*. For this purpose we have carried out cDNA–RNA annealing reactions under less stringent conditions (lower temperature, higher salt). In experiments conducted to date we have established that

Table 4. C-type virus and MPMV cDNA annealing with MCF-7 RNA[a]

		% Hybrid formation at $C_r t = 10^4$ Source of RNA			
Probe number	Source of viral cDNA	RLV	MPMV (NC37)	Balb/cfc3H primary cells	MCF+ cells
C-1	RLV (Plasma)	98	NT	11	0
C-2	RLV (Plasma)	96	NT	4	2
C-4	RLV (Plasma)	92	2	16	2
P-3	MPMV (NC37)	ND	89	1	2

[a]Viral cDNAs were prepared according to the methods in the legend for Figure 5. Single-stranded (> 90% digestible by S_1 nuclease) DNA products of reverse transcriptase reactions elicited from isopycnically banded C-type viruses were hybridized to RNA extracted from various cell or viruses. Hybridization mixtures contained 500 cpm of DNA, unlabeled RNA, and 0.4 M NaCl, 0.025 M Tris-HCl (pH 7.4), and 0.001 M EDTA. Incubation temperature was 68°; reaction time was 66 hr. The extent of annealing of labeled virus DNA to RNA was measured by enzymatic (S_1) digestion of unhybridized DNA according to the methods of Ref. 32. Percent hybridization values are those with only background (scintillation counter) subtracted. Less than 5% hybridization may be considered nonspecific with these probes. RNAs are: 70 S RNA from Rauscher Leukemia virus (RLV); 50–70 S RNA from MPMV; primary MuMTV-induced Balb/cfc3H mammary tumor RNA; and MCF-7 RNA from which 734B was obtained. $C_r t$ values of 10^4 are saturation values for all RLV and MPMV sDNA-RNA hybridizations.

Table 5. MuMTV cDNA annealing with MCF-7 RNA[a]

		% Hybrid formation at $C_r t = 10^4$ source of RNA			
Probe number	Source of viral cDNA	3T3	Balb/cfc3H	MCF-7	H. placenta
B-10	RIII milk	2	96	6	3
B-19	RIII milk	6	92(66°)	37(63°)	5
B-26	RIII milk	5	89	4	2
B-68	Balb/cfc3H	4	96	29(63°)	6

[a]Viral cDNAs and cell RNAs were prepared as described in legend to Figure 5. Single-stranded MuMTV cDNAs were annealed to the cell RNAs shown under the conditions established in Ref. 32 (Figure 5). Numbers in parentheses represent T_m values for denaturation of DNA–RNA hybrids formed at $C_r t = 10^4$. Temperature denaturations were conducted in 0.0. M Tris (pH 8.1) and analyzed by S_1 nuclease digestion of unhybridized DNA (32). The same source of MCF-7 RNA (122T) was used for all hybridizations shown.

some of the MuMTV cDNAs that did not anneal under more stringent conditions do anneal with MCF$^+$ RNA at 50°C in 50% formamide at a $C_r t$ of 10^4. These MuMTV cDNAs did not anneal significantly with human liver or placental RNA, nor did MuLV (Rauscher) cDNA anneal with MCF$^+$ RNA under those conditions. MPMV cDNA likewise did not react with MCF-7 RNA under these more permissive conditions. Thus, MuMTV and 734B appear to be related, with considerable homology between their nucleotide sequences; however, significant mismatching occurs in the hybrids, indicating a significant divergence in the genomes of the two viruses. Quantitative studies using MCF$^+$ RNA to competitively inhibit hybrid formation between MuMTV cDNA and RNA are in progress to elucidate the true genetic relationship between the two viruses.

IV.   DNA POLYMERASES ASSOCIATED WITH 734B

Two DNA polymerases have been identified in 734B preparations. One of these functions as a reverse transcriptase in endogenous reactions; the other functions as a DNA templated DNA polymerase.

The 734B reverse transcriptase has been characterized by the fact that the endogenous reaction using NP40 activated virions is sensitive to ribonuclease and that endogenous heteropolymeric RNA is used as *template* to synthesize DNA in a reaction requiring all four nucleoside triphosphates (20). This was established by denaturing the DNA–RNA hybrid product (23) and demonstrating that the DNA separated from the RNA under the denaturation conditions (20).

The exact size of the RNA serving as template in the reverse transcriptase reaction has not been established. That the RNA is of high molecular weight is suggested by the fact that DNA–RNA hybrids, identified in "simultaneous detection assays," exhibit molecular weights of $10–12 \times 10^6$ and $3–5 \times 10^6$ (20), and by analysis of native and denatured products of high and low molecular weight in CsSO$_4$ equilibrium density gradients. With the latter, we have established that a minimum of 40% of the denaturable DNA–RNA hybrid product can be recovered from the high molecular weight ($> 20S$) region of 5–20% "simultaneous detection" rate zonal sucrose gradients. Direct demonstration that the high molecular weight template RNA is the $10–12 \times 10^6$-dalton material has been difficult because of the relatively small amount of RNA in the RNA–DNA product (20).

Further characterization of the enzyme with respect to its response to various synthetic template-primers and its sensitivity to neutralization with antisera prepared against nonhuman viral polymerases requires additional purification of the enzyme. Preliminary data suggest that microsomal preparations of MCF$^+$ cells provide a richer source of 734B enzyme than do cell-free particles. Efforts are currently underway to purify the enzyme from this source.

Another DNA polymerizing activity has been identified in several gradient-purified preparations of MCF-7 culture supernatants. This activity (DDDP) can be distinguished from the bona fide reverse transcriptase activity (RDDP) by its sensitivity to low concentrations of actinomycin D, and its relative insensitivity to ribonuclease (Table 6). In addition, a 20- to 100-fold stimulation of [³H]thymidine triphosphate incorporation has been observed with an activated DNA template (Table 6). Since the enzyme has been observed under conditions where neither 734B RDDP enzyme nor marker polypeptides could be identified (cf. Table 2), the DDDP is likely not associated with 734B particles, but rather with cell constituents contaminating 1.16–1.18 g/cm³ gradient bands.

The RDDP can be distinguished from the DDDP by the nature of the endogenous DNA product as well as the criteria just described. Differences in the nucleotide sequence nature of the products of the two reactions are described below.

V.   NUCLEOTIDE SEQUENCE NATURE OF
DNA SYNTHESIZED BY 734B DNA POLYMERASES
AND SPECULATION ON THE ORIGIN OF THE VIRUS

DNA products of the actinomycin D sensitive DDDP reaction associated with 734B have not annealed with any of the human or mouse cytoplasmic or viral RNAs used to date. This includes MCF-7 RNA, Balb/cfc3H tumor RNA, and AMV, MuLV, and MuMTV viral RNA. Stable hybrids, however, have been formed between these DNAs and MCF-7 cellular DNA but only at high $C_o t$ values (Table 6). These DNA products appear, therefore, to represent cell genes not transcribed in sufficient number to be detected in the DNA–RNA hybridizations.

Table 6. DNA polymerases associated with 734B

Source of enzyme[a]	Enzyme designation[b]	Relative activity[c]	Sensitivity to actinomycin D[d]	Sensitivity to RNAase[e]	Utilization of "Activated" DNA[f]	Nature of RNA product MCF+ RNA[g] Anneal with	MCF+ DNA[h] Anneal with
p=1.16–1.18	RDDP	+	No	Yes	No	Yes	Yes
p=1.20–1.21	DDDP	+++	Yes	No	Yes	No	Yes

[a]Particles from MCF+ culture supernatants, with densities corresponding to those shown, were pooled from sucrose gradients and pelleted. Endogenous polymerase reactions were elicited by addition of 0.25% NP40 in the reaction system described (20). dT_{12-18} (30 μg/ml) was included in all reactions.

[b]RDDP, RNA directed DNA polymerase; DDDP, DNA directed DD polymerase.

[c]Activity is compared to MuMTV RDDP activity (4+) at equivalent viral DNA concentration.

[d]Actinomycin D (100 μg/ml), added to NP40 activated particles eliminated DDDP activity ($>$ 85% diminution); RDDP activity was unaffected.

[e]Pancreatic RNAase (15 μg/ml) was added to NP40 activated particles for 10 min at 37°C before addition of nucleoside triphosphates (20).

[f]Calf thymus DNA, nicked by incubations with DNAase II as described (27).

[g]Hybridization was determined by cDNA–RNA reaction in 0.4 M NaCl as described in the legend for Figure 5.

[h]Hybridization was determined by hydroxyapatite chromatography as described in the legend for Figure 6.

The DNA products of the bona fide 734B reverse transcriptase reactions have also been annealed with nuclear DNA from several sources as well as with RNA from a variety of cell types. The primary objective of DNA–DNA annealing studies to date has been to establish the species of origin for 734B. The primary objective of cDNA–RNA hybridizations has been to establish the specificity of the cDNAs as probes for 734B in the DNA–DNA hybridizations.

On the basis of annealing characteristics under stringent hybridization conditions (0.4 M NaCl, 68°) with MCF^+ RNA, MCF^- RNA, human liver RNA, and human breast tumor RNA, two classes of 734B cDNAs have been identified: class 1 cDNAs anneal to high levels with normal liver RNA as well as MCF^+ RNA (Table 7). These cDNAs also anneal to high levels with MCF^- RNA and a breast tumor RNA. Class 2 cDNAs anneal with MCF^+ RNA to greater than 60% levels at a $C_r t$ of 10^4. Under these same conditions, hybridizations with liver RNA do not occur (Table 7). Hybridization with MCF^- RNA has not exceeded 8% for class 2 cDNAs at $C_r t$ values of 10^4, while significant hybridization was observed with RNA from a human breast tumor (Table 7). While insufficient amounts of class 2 DNA have been available to date to determine the T_m values for these hybrids, annealing under the stringent conditions of these experiments suggests a high degree of bona fide base pairing in the hybrids.

We have used these class 2 cDNAs in DNA–DNA annealing, using vast excesses (by weight) of nuclear DNAs. The results of these experiments are shown in Figure 6. At $C_o t$ values beyond 100, only human placental nuclear DNA formed hybrids with class 2

Table 7. Specificity of 734B cDNAs, % hybrid formation at $C_r t = 10^4$, source of RNA[a]

cDNA preparation	MCF-7^+	MCF-7^-	H. liver	Human breast tumor no. 109
A—40 (Class 1)	65	26	40	33
A—63 (Class 1)	70	39	51	44
A—59 (Class 2)	87	2	1	37
A—68 (Class 2)	75	8	2	42

[a]734B cDNAs were prepared as for MuMTV cDNAs (in Mg^{++} containing buffers; cf. Figure 5). Hybridizations were conducted at 68° in buffers 0.4 M with respect to Na^+ ion (see legend to Figure 5).

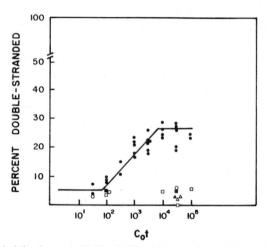

Figure 6. Hybridization of 734B cDNA with nuclear DNA of cells from several species. Nuclei were extracted from tissue cells and DNA was extracted from nuclei as recommended in Ref. 25. cDNA-nuclear DNA hybridizations were conducted in 0.4 M sodium phosphate buffers using 400 cpm of cDNA and 1 mg of nuclear DNA. $C_o t$ values were calculated as recommended in Ref. 8 and were varied experimentally by varying time of incubation at 68°C. Percent hybridization was determined by hydroxyapatite chromatography in 0.15 M NaCl (25). The data shown are the material that eluted from columns between 88° and 96°C or "perfectly paired" Watson-Crick hybrids. 734B cDNA was annealed with *Bacillus subtilis* DNA as a specificity control in the hybridization; these percent hybridization (~ 2%) with this DNA has been subtracted from the values shown. Class 2 cDNA was annealed with human placental DNA (●), cat liver DNA (○), bovine thymus DNA (■), mouse liver DNA (□), rhesus monkey liver DNA (▲), and hamster DNA (△).

cDNAs. Maximum hybrid formation (28%) was achieved with human placental DNA with a plateau at $C_o t$ values between 10^4 and 10^5. These data suggest that those sequences in human cell DNA that hybridized to 734B cDNA are probably repeated in the genome rather than infrequently represented (13). Bovine, feline, mouse, hamster, and rhesus monkey DNAs did not anneal with class 2 cDNAs at $C_o t$ values of 10^4–10^5. The fact that 734B cDNA (class 2) did not anneal with mouse DNA offers compelling proof that 734B is not identical with MuMTV. Identity between 734B and endogenous viruses of the other four species tested is equally unlikely.

The extent to which 734B nucleotide sequences are represented in normal human cells and, in turn, the species of origin for 734B, depends largely on two considerations: (1) the specificity of the class 2 cDNAs used in the DNA–DNA reassociation experiments and (2) the extent to which the 734B genome is represented by the cDNAs used. The fact that the cDNAs used in the DNA–DNA reassociation experiments did not anneal specifically to human liver or placental RNAs but did anneal to MCF^+ RNA at a rate 10–30 times that of MCF^- RNA ($C_rt_{1/2}$ of $10^{3.2}$ versus $C_rt_{1/2}$ of $10^{4-4.6}$) suggests that these cDNAs are specific for 734B RNA. If the class 2 cDNAs were complementary to human cell (e.g., ribosomal) RNA, we would have expected substantial annealing of class 2 cDNAs with liver or placental RNA and also substantial annealing of the cDNAs to nonhuman DNAs (13). This was not observed for class 2 cDNAs. It should be noted, however, that the most rigorous demonstration of the specificity of 734B class 2 cDNA requires availability of hybridization data with high molecular weight RNA extracted from cell-free 734B and RNA from normal breast epithelium.

The results of a preliminary study in which maximum hybridization for a 734B cDNA (class 2) at a C_ot of 10^4 was 31% with human placental DNA (C_ot $10^3 = 31\%$) and 53% with MCF^+ DNA (C_ot $10^3 = 28\%$) suggest that the cDNAs may represent more of the 734B genome than the approximately 30% of *repetitive* sequences present in human placental DNA. This, in turn, suggests incomplete representation of the 734B genome in nuclear DNA of normal placental cells.

The additional sequences detected by the cDNA in MCF^+ cells at a C_ot of 10^4 probably represent infrequent 734B sequences. The question whether these infrequent sequences are also present in nuclear DNA of malignant human breast cells is being actively pursued.

Our results show that annealing between 734B cDNAs and cell DNAs conducted under stringent hybridization conditions occurred only with human and not with nonhuman (including one simian) nuclear DNA. These data suggest an origin for some 734B genes from human DNA. The question of whether 734B was actually generated indigenously from human chromosomal DNA or was inserted into human cell DNA by horizontal transmission followed by genetic divergence is a question that can only be resolved by more extensive hybridization studies with 734B cDNAs and a spectrum of cell DNA selected on the basis of mouse/human phylogeny.

86   McGrath et al.

LITERATURE CITED

1. Achong, B., P. Mansell, M. Epstein, and P. Clifford (1971). J. Nat. Cancer Inst. 46:299–307.
2. Ahmed, M., S. Mayyasi, H. Chopra, J. Zelljadt, and E. Jensen (1971). J. Nat. Cancer Inst. 46:1325–1330.
3. Arnold, W., H. Soule, and J. Russo (1975). In Vitro 10:356.
4. August, J. T., D. Bolognesi, E. Fleissner, R. Gilden, and R. C. Nowinski (1974). Virology 60:595–601.
5. Axel, R., S. Gulati, and S. Spiegelman (1972). Proc. Nat. Acad. Sci., U.S.A. 69:3133–3137.
6. Benveniste, R. and G. Todaro (1973). Proc. Nat. Acad. Sci., U.S.A. 70:3316–3320.
7. Bernhard, W. (1973). *In:* Ultrastructure of Animal Viruses and Bacteriophages, J. Dalton, and F. Hagenau, Eds., p. 283. Academic Press, New York.
8. Britten, R. (1969). Carnegie Inst. Wash. Yearbook 68:378–386.
9. Brooks, S., E. Locke, and H. Soule (1973). J. Biol. Chem. 248:6251–6253.
10. Buehring, G. and A. Hackett (1974). J. Nat. Cancer Inst. 53:621–629.
11. Chopra, H. and M. Mason (1970). Cancer Res. 30:2081–2084.
12. Gallo, R., R. Gallagher, N. Miller, H. Mondal, W. Saxinger, R. Mayer, R. Smith, and D. Gillespie (1975). Cold Spring Harbor Symp. Quant. Biol. 39:933–963.
13. Gillespie, D. and R. C. Gallo (1974). Science 188:802–811.
14. Green, R. and D. Bolognesi (1974). Anal. Biochem. 57:108–117.
15. Greenwood, F. C., W. M. Hunter, and J. S. Clover (1963). Biochem. J. 89:114–123.
16. Ilyin, K., I. Irlin, A. Bykovsky, Z. Spure, G. Miller, U. Abenova, and V. Zhdanov (1974). Cancer 34:532–538.
17. Ilyin, K., A. Bykovsky, and V. Zhdanov (1973). Cancer 32:89–96.
18. Maizel, J. (1969). *In:* Fundamental Techniques in Virology, K. Habel and N. P. Salzman, Eds. Academic Press, New York.
19. McGrath, C. M. (1971). J. Nat. Cancer Inst. 47:455–467.
20. McGrath, C., P. Grant, H. Soule, T. Glancy, and M. Rich (1974). Nature 252:247–250.
21. Nelson-Rees, W., R. Flandermeyer, and P. Hawthrone (1974). Science 184:1093–1096.
22. Parks, W., R. Howk, E. Scolnick, S. Oroszlan, and R. Gilden (1974). J. Virol. 13:1200–1210.
23. Reitz, M., J. Abrell, C. Tracnov, and R. Gallo (1972). Biochem. Biophys. Res. Commun. 49:30–38.
24. Rose, H. and C. McGrath (1975). Science 190:673–675.
25. Ruprecht, R., N. Goodman, and S. Spiegelman (1973). Proc. Nat. Acad. Sci. U.S.A. 70:1437–1441.

26. Russo, J. H. Soule, C. McGrath, and M. Rich (1975). J. Nat. Cancer Inst., in press.

27. Schlabach, A., A. Fridlender, A. Bolden, and A. Weissbach (1971). Biochem. Biophys. Res. Commun. 44:879–885.

28. Soule, H., J. Vasquez, A. Long, S. Albert, and M. Brennan (1973). J. Nat. Cancer Inst. 51:1409–1416.

29. Strand, M. and J. T. August (1973). J. Biol. Chem. 248:5627–5633.

30. Teramoto, Y., M. Puentes, L. J. T. Young, and R. D. Cardiff (1974). J. Virol. 13:411–418.

31. Teramoto, Y. and R. Cardiff (1975). Proc. Am. Assoc. Cancer Res. 16:133.

32. Varmus, H., N. Quintrell, E. Medeiros, J. M. Bishop, R. Nowinski, and N. Sarkar (1973). J. Mol. Biol. 79:663–679.

33. Voyles, B., H. Soule, and C. McGrath (1974). In Vitro 10:389.

CHAPTER 5

Herpesvirus Antigens and Cell-Mediated Immunity in Cervical Cancer

L. Aurelian, B. C. Strand,
R. P. Jacobs, R. B. Bell, and M. F. Smith

I. INTRODUCTION

Although herpesviruses destroy the cells in which they multiply in vitro, they are notorious for their ability to persist in the infected host in a latent state, i.e., without causing clinically obvious disease. The products of virus expression during latency, their regulation and their respective role in modulating host immune responses are not yet clearly understood. Also, herpesviruses, and particularly HSV-2, have been associated with cancer (29, 30, 36) and thus the ability to confer upon infected cells uncontrolled replication and immortality. An antigen designated AG-4, made only in infected cells, has been associated with active tumor growth (2). The exact nature of this antigen (viral or cellular), and the virus–host cell interactions resulting in its expression may play a significant role in cancer progression or control.

High levels of circulating antibody to the various antigens of HSV-1 and HSV-2 are generally observed in most populations and

Studies supported by Contract NO-1-CP-33345 and NO-1-CP-43330 of the Special Virus Cancer Program, National Cancer Institute.

persist for long periods. These represent various immunoglobulins and possibly even allotypes, differing in properties and under different control (35). Their presence in the infected host together with various populations of memory and effector cells possibly regulated independently of the humoral responses, must be interpreted in terms of the multitude of herpesvirus antigens (type, common, or specific), their expression during clinical disease (productive, latent, or neoplastic), their role in the modulation of immune responses, and the probable in vivo interaction of all these factors.

The purpose of this chapter is to present these problems in light of the information available to date, and to point to avenues of research that might furnish answers to at least some of the questions raised.

II.   HSV-2 AND SQUAMOUS CANCER OF THE HUMAN CERVIX

The available evidence associating HSV-2 with cervical neoplasia has been reviewed (30, 36), and may be summarized as follows: First, seroepidemiologic studies indicate that patients with cervical cancer have antibody to HSV-2 at a much higher frequency than controls that are matched for age, race, and socioeconomic class (4, 29, 36). It is of particular significance that the results of the various studies done on different populations agree in conclusions that associate HSV-2 with cervical cancer (29), despite the large number of experimental variables including serologic assay, virus prototypes, and epidemiologic design. Second, cervical tumor cells contain HSV-2 DNA, viral RNA, and antigens, both structural and nonstructural (1, 2, 5, 11, 15, 17, 21). In terms of the etiology hypothesis, it should be pointed out that active tumor growth is associated with the synthesis of a HSV-2 antigen, designated AG-4 (2, 3). Third, HSV-2 can transform cells in vitro (18, 40), and at least some of the transformed clones cause tumors in animals (40). Finally, HSV-2 has recently been shown to cause atypia in cebus monkeys (39).

Assuming that HSV-2 causes cancer of the cervix, three questions arise. First, does the virus cause the transformation of the cell from normal to neoplastic or does it act upon the transformed cell as a selective agent leading to the establishment of a neoplastic clone? Second, is the virus ever latent in the cell before transforming it? Finally, since the stress conditions capable of inducing recurrent productive disease occur even after transformation, why is it they no longer induce virus replication and cell death?

The role played by HSV-2 in the original transformation of the cell it has infected cannot be unequivocally determined. In animal models, in vitro transformation by inactivated HSV-2 (and HSV-1) has been reported. With one exception, transformed cells contain type C virus genome, raising questions as to the exact involvement of HSV (18, 40). Also, inactivated virus fails to induce cellular DNA synthesis (34). There still is some controversy as to the criteria acceptable for transformation. With the exception of one oncogenic clone, HSV-2 induced transformation has been defined as the presence of virus antigens and virions in the cells in the absence of infection (13, 40).

In most human cancers, the in vivo stage equivalent to in vitro transformation either does not exist or at least has not been detected. Precancerous lesions of cervical carcinoma are easily identifiable and it is conceivable that atypia is an in vivo counterpart of in vitro transformation. Evidence that HSV-2 causes cellular atypia in man is: (a) infection with the virus precedes even its earliest detectable form (4); (b) women with cytologic evidence of HSV-2 infection develop cervical atypia at a higher frequency than uninfected subjects (37), (c) using the same criteria as those used for most in vitro transformants, HSV-2 antigens are present in the tumor cells from 80% of cervical atypia cases (5, 17), and (d) HSV-2 appears to cause atypia in cebus monkeys (39) and the virus was isolated from cervical tumor cells in culture (6).

It is possible that only cells maintaining the appropriate defective genome become transformed. This interpretation predicts that (a) functional and defective viral genomes can be maintained in a latent state by cells other than neurons, (b) defective virions are produced during productive infection, and (c) defective genomes can transform cells. Bronson et al. (9) have shown that defective DNA is produced and incorporated into virions in cells infected at a high multiplicity of infection. It is not clear whether defectiveness represents presence of some, but not all, viral DNA sequences, cellular DNA (pseudovirions), or modified viral DNA. In support of this interpretation is the presence in a cervical tumor of only a fragment of the HSV-2 DNA (15). Complete HSV particles in 2 of 14 human invasive cervical tumors (22) does not necessarily preclude this interpretation. However, it suggests that defectiveness is not due to the absence of some of the nucleic acid sequences. Another possibility, not necessarily discounted by the susceptibility of cervical tumor cells to reinfection with HSV-2 (6), is that transformed cells contain host-to-virus factors ("repressors") that block virus multiplication. Absence of viral DNA in human cervical cancer biopsies is easily explained by the paucity of tumor cells (estimated as 1 in 10,000) in such material. Absence of viral DNA in cells transformed in vitro is more difficult to explain, particularly because the cells contain virus particles (11, 41).

Precancerous lesions (atypia and carcinoma in situ) can regress or they can progress to invasive cervical cancer (27, 32). The isolation of infectious HSV-2 from cultured cells obtained from a precancerous lesion (6) and the observation that it had persisted according to the predictions of the static-state hypothesis (44), favor the interpretation that HSV-2 is latent in the cells it transforms. In order to prove unequivocally that latency is a precursor step to transformation, it is necessary to establish bona fide latent cultures in vitro, define the operative mechanisms that will transform these cells, determine whether transformation requires the presence and maintenance of the same sequences of viral DNA as those present in latency, and show that all cancers associated with this virus contain at least some of the same set of DNA sequences.

A.   Association of an Antigen (AG-4) with Active Tumor Growth

Possibly most significant from the point of view of virus causation are the recent data indicating the presence in cervical cancer biopsies of an antigen (AG-4) that is also HSV-2 induced (2). This antigen, assayed by complement fixation is not present in biopsied sections of a normal cervix (2, 3). The significance of the antigen is that its presence appears to reflect active tumor growth. As summarized in Table 1, the prevalence of antibody to AG-4 is significantly higher in patients with invasive carcinoma (85%) than in a matched control group (12%) and it correlates with the gradation expected of cervical cancer (atypia, 43%; in situ, 65%) (27, 32). Most significantly, AG-4 antibody is absent in patients with cervical cancer successfully treated prior to blood collection, but reappears in those with a recurrent neoplastic disease, indicating that virus expression is necessary for tumor development. Neutralizing antibody to HSV-2, on the other hand, is uniformly prevalent in both cancer patients and controls and is not affected by therapy.

Herpesvirus Antigens and Immunity 93

Table 1. Presence of antibody to AG-4 in cancer patients and controls

Group	No. Tested	Positive for AG-4[a]		Positive for AG-H		Positive for HSV-2[b]	
		No.	%	No.	%	No.	%
Atypia	7	3	43	0	0	7	100
Matched controls	7	0	0	0	0	4	57
In situ	20	13	65	0	0	19	95
Matched controls	20	1	5	0	0	10	50
Invasive	34	29	85	0	0	34	100
Matched controls	34	4	12	5	15	24	71
Treated invasive cancer	26	0	0	0	0	26	100
Recurrent cancer	7	6	86	0	0	7	100

[a]Complement fixation assay.
[b]Neutralization assay.

The experiments described below were designed to investigate the nature (viral or cellular) of AG-4. The rationale for the experimental design was 2-fold. First, it was argued that comparison of the polypeptides in cell extracts capable of fixing complement with AG-4 positive sera, to those in extracts deprived of AG-4 activity, may serve in identifying those polypeptides specifically associated with the AG-4 antigen. Second, simultaneous comparison of these polypeptides to those obtained from purified virions would help in identifying the AG-4 associated polypeptides as virion proteins. In view of the observation that HSV-1 also codes for 24 nonstructural polypeptides (25) and considering the possibility that AG-4 may be a nonstructural virion protein, we also studied cells infected with HSV-2 for various time intervals. The criteria whereby an infected cell polypeptide (ICP) was accepted as virus-specific were the same as those used by Honess and Roizman (25) and essentially consisted of the kinetics of polypeptide synthesis, their relative abundance, immunoprecipitation by specific antisera, and variability associated with different virus strains.

B.   Kinetics of AG-4 Synthesis

Two-day-old monolayer cultures of HEp-2 cells were infected with 0.4 plaque-forming units (PFU) of HSV-2/cell and incubated at 37°C for 1 hr. At that time (0 hr), the inoculum was aspirated, and the cells were washed with phosphate-buffered saline (PBS) and overlayed with maintenance medium consisting of medium 199 (Grand Island Biological) with 1% calf serum. At the time intervals indicated in Figure 1, samples consisting of two replicate cultures were recovered and assayed for infectious virus and for AG-4 activity using a patient serum (No. 7) previously shown to fix complement with AG-4, although it did not have measurable antibody to HSV-2. Synthesis of AG-4 starts at 4 hr after infection, 1 hr before virus progeny is first observed, and proceeds at an optimal rate until 9 hr. At 18 hr, when the yield of virus is 3.5 PFU/cell, AG-4 activity is not detectable. Synthesis of AG-4 is not affected by cell age or clone history of the HEp-2 cells. AG-H prepared in parallel does not fix complement. The data indicate that AG-4 synthesis does not correlate with virion formation in complete agreement with the serologic results (Table 1) showing that antibody to AG-4 is distinct from neutralizing antibody. Absence of AG-4 activity, 18 hr after infection, when virus yields are optimal, suggests that AG-4 is (a)

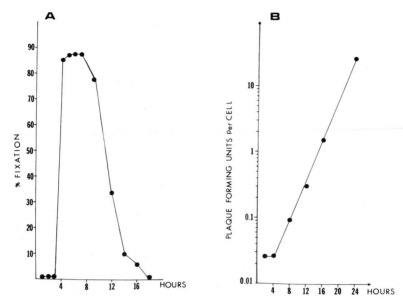

Figure 1. *A*, kinetics of AG-4 synthesis in HEp-2 cells infected with HSV-2 (G strain). Samples collected at each time interval were assayed against AG-4 positive and negative sera by complement fixation. The AG-4 positive serum used in this study did not have measurable HSV-2 antibody. Fixation was not observed with the AG-4 negative serum. *B*, formation of HSV-2 in simultaneously infected replicate HEp-2 cultures.

a host protein induced by virus infection, (b) a nonstructural viral protein made early in infection, or (c) a structural viral protein, located inside the virion and made in relatively lower abundance after 9 hr postinfection.

C.   Relationship of AG-4 to Virion Surface Antigens

Experiments were designed to determine the ability of AG-4 to block the neutralizing potential of (a) rabbit antiserum to HSV-2 (Ra-2) and (b) two human sera, Nos. 142 and 145, obtained from cervical cancer cases and respectively containing antibody to HSV-2 alone or to both HSV-2 and HSV-1. The results, summarized in Figure 2, indicate that various concentrations of AG-4 have no effect on the neutralizing capacity of serum 142. Identical results were obtained with sera No. 145 and Ra-2, further confirming that AG-4 is antigenically distinct from virion surface antigens.

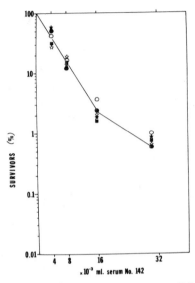

Figure 2. Inability of AG-4 to block the HSV-2 neutralizing power of human serum No. 142.

D.   AG-4, a Cell Surface Antigen

The search for the cellular location of AG-4 was made possible by the observation that antibody to AG-4 is IgM (7) and by the adaptation of the anticomplement immunofluorescence (ACIF) test (43). Various dilutions of IgM fractions were mixed with a HSV negative human serum serving as a source of complement, and used to stain HEp-2 cells infected with HSV-2 for 4 and 24 hr. These time intervals were selected because they represented the time of synthesis of AG-4 and virus, respectively.

IgM from all AG-4 positive and two of four AG-4 negative sera produced surface granular fluorescence (Figure 3) on both 4- and 24-hr-infected cells. The surface nature of this fluorescence was confirmed by staining unfixed cells in suspension. For most sera antibody titers, calculated as the highest staining IgM dilution, were similar for the 4- and 24-hours-infected cells.

There are virus-coded glycoproteins on infected cell membranes and virion envelopes (20). However, based on the inability of AG-4 to block serum neutralizing potential and the kinetics of its synthesis, it must be considered different from these glycoproteins. IgM fractions were adsorbed prior to ACIF assays with (a) 24-hr-

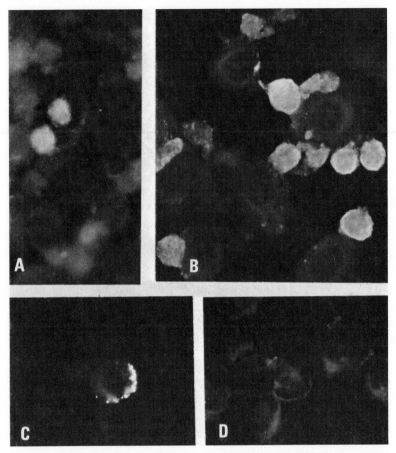

Figure 3. ACIF staining of HEp-2 cells infected with HSV-2 for 4 hrs. (× 437) *A*, fixed infected cells stained with IgM from serum No. 17 adsorbed with HSV-2; *B*, fixed infected cells stained with unadsorbed IgM from serum No. 17; *C*, unfixed infected cells stained with IgM from serum No. 63; *D*, fixed uninfected cells stained with unadsorbed IgM from serum No. 17.

infected HEp-2 cells, (b) virus pelleted by centrifugation for 1.5 hr in a Spinco SW 27 rotor at 25,000 rpm, or (c) 4-hr-infected HEp-2 cells. The results (Table 2) indicate that following adsorbtion with virions or 24-hr-infected cells, the IgM from AG-4 positive sera become negative for 24-hr-infected cells, but maintain their ability to stain a small number (2–5%) of HEp-2 cells infected with HSV-2 for 4 hr. IgM from AG-4 negative sera no longer stain 24- or 4-hr-infected cells. Following adsorption with cells infected for

Table 2. ACIF staining of HSV-2 infected HEp-2 cells with immunoglobulins adsorbed with HSV-2

Immunoglobulin	ACIF of HSV-2 infected with HEp-2 cells	
	4 hr	24 hr
25 IgM		
Unadsorbed (1/4)	+ (9%)	+ (3%)
Adsorbed with		
HEp-2 cells	+ (9%)	+ (2%)
HEp/HSV-2/4 hr	+ (5%)	—
HEp/HSV-2/4 hr	—	—
8 IgM, 10 IgM		
Unadsorbed (1/2)	+ (6%)	+ (2%)
Adsorbed with		
HEp-2 cells	+ (4%)	+ (2%)
HEp/HSV-2/24 hr	—	—
17 IgM		
Unadsorbed (1/10)	+ (16%)	+ (12%)
Unadsorbed (1/40)	+ (0.1%)	+ (30%)
Diluted 1/10 and		
Adsorbed with		
HEp-2 cells	+ (12%)	+ (12%)
Pelleted HSV-2	+ (2%)	—
HEp/HSV-2/4 hr	—	—
13 IgM		
Unadsorbed (1/10)	+ (6.7%)	+ (10%)
Adsorbed with		
HEp-2 cells	+ (8%)	+ (9%)
Pelleted HSV-2	+ (3.5%)	—
HEp/HSV-2/4 hr	—	—
160 IgM		
Unadsorbed (1/4)	+ (4.1)%	+ (4.8%)
Adsorbed with		
HEp-2 cells	+ (4%)	+ (3%)
Pelleted HSV-2	+ (1.7%)	—
HEp/HSV-2/4 hr	—	—
63 IgM		
Unadsorbed (1/10)	+ (10%)	+ (40%)
Adsorbed with		
HEp-2 cells	+ (10%)	+ (40%)
Pelleted HSV-2	+ (3%)	—
HEp/HSV-2/4 hr	+ (1%)	—

Table 2. continued

Immunoglobulin	ACIF of HSV-2 infected with HEp-2 cells	
	4 hr	24 hr
63 IgG		
Unadsorbed (1/80)	+ (12%)	+ (30%)
Adsorbed with		
HEp-2 cells	+ (15%)	+ (30%)
Pelleted HSV-2	−	−
HEp-2/HSV-2/4 hr	−	−
12 IgG		
Unadsorbed (1/80)	+ (10%)	+ (22%)
Adsorbed with		
HEp-2 cells	+ (7.8%)	+ (25%)
Pelleted HSV-2	−	−
HEp-2/HSV-2/4 hr	−	−
HEp-2/HSV-2/24 hr	−	−
25 IgG		
Unadsorbed (1/40)	+ (5%)	+ (10%)
Adsorbed with		
HEp-2 cells	+ (5%)	+ (8%)
Pelleted HSV-2	−	−
HEp-2/HSV-2/4 hr	−	−

4 hr, IgM from both AG-4 positive and negative sera do not stain 4- or 24-hr-infected cells. It may be concluded that the ability of IgM to fix complement with AG-4 correlates with its ACIF staining potential for 2–5% of the 4-hr-infected cells and that AG-4 is located on the cell surface. However, unequivocal evidence to this effect must await the preparation of monospecific sera.

E. HSV-2 Virion Proteins

In order to determine the number, electrophoretic mobility, and hence, the molecular weights, of the virus specific proteins in the purified virions, HSV-2 (G strain) was prepared in HEp-2 cells labeled with [^{35}S]methionine between 6 and 24 hr postinfection and purified according to the method of Spear and Roizman (48). Briefly, packed cells in 1 mM phosphate buffer (pH 7.4) were disrupted with four strokes of a Dounce homogenizer and sufficient 60% (w/w) sucrose was added to yield a final concentration of

0.25 M. The cytoplasm was separated from the nuclei by centrifugation at 1,500 rpm for 10 min in a PR-2 International Refrigerated Centrifuge and the cytoplasmic extract centrifuged on two consecutive dextran-10 gradients. Such procedures were shown to separate virions from soluble proteins and most cellular membrane vesicles that remain on top of the gradient, and from aggregates of virions, cytoplasmic organelles, and large debris that pellet. Specifically, 2-ml samples of cytoplasm were layered onto 36-ml dextran-10 gradients (1.04–1.09 g/ml) made in 1 mM phosphate buffer and centrifuged at 20,000 rpm for 1 hr in a Spinco SW 27 rotor. The virions found in a diffuse light scattering band just above the middle of the tube were collected, made 0.5 M with respect to urea, and sonicated for 5 sec to dissociate aggregates of virus particles and host membrane vesicles. Following dilution with 0.01 M Tris buffer (pH 7.4), the suspensions were centrifuged at 25,000 rpm for 1.5 hr in a Spinco SW 27 rotor. Immediately before electrophoresis, the proteins in the virus pellets were denatured and solubilized by the addition of small volumes of 0.05 M Tris-hydrochloride (pH 7.0), 2% sodium dodecyl sulfate (SDS), 5% β-mercaptoethanol, and 0.005% bromphenol blue followed by boiling for 2 min. The solubilized proteins (100–150 μg) were subjected to electrophoresis on acrylamide gels employing the discontinuous buffer system modified by the inclusion of SDS (12). The 8.5% concentration of acrylamide was chosen because it gave the best overall resolution of virus proteins (48). Autoradiography of gel cylinders longitudinally cut in half was done according to the method described by Fairbanks et al. (14).

The yield and purity of the virion preparations were determined by negative-stain electron microscopy and by estimates of the recovery of infectivity and virus-specific label. The virus band from the first dextran gradient consisted almost exclusively of intact enveloped nucleocapsids with very rare membrane contaminants, which appeared to diminish further after the second gradient. Plaque-forming units (PFU)/cpm ratios were 50 times higher in the first gradient than in the crude homogenate (Table 3). Approximately a 2-fold improvement in virus purification over the first gradient was observed during the second.

Analyses of the virion proteins by autoradiography following solubilization and electrophoresis are highly reproducible. There are 24 virus-specific proteins in the virion designated as VP 1–VP 24 (Figure 4).

Table 3. Purification of HSV-2 virions: Recovery of infectivity[a] and virus-specific label

	PFU/cpm	Fold purification
Cell suspension	8.85	1
Cytoplasmic fraction	47.4	5.35
Nuclear fraction	11.0	1.24
Virus band (1st dextran)	456	51.3

[a]Correction is not made for the losses in infectivity occuring during centrifugation. Assuming such losses are due to biologic changes without causing significant physical modifications, a further 2-fold increase in purification can be calculated.

Molecular weights of the viral proteins were estimated by determining their migration rates relative to proteins whose molecular weights were well characterized (47, 51). For the standard proteins smaller than 100,000 daltons, a plot of logarithm of molecular weight versus relative migration rate yielded a straight line. In 8.5% acrylamide, the standard proteins larger than 100,000 daltons migrate faster than would be expected if they had obeyed the inverse logarithmic function between molecular weight and relative migration rate; however, a smooth curved line was drawn to fit the points from which molecular weights are estimated (48). The relative mobilities of the protein standards and of viral proteins in the gels are shown in Figure 5. The average molecular weights range from 16,000 to 250,000. These results agree with those described by Spear and Roizman (48) for HSV-1, both with respect to the number of virion proteins and the range of molecular weights. On the other hand, as reported by Honess et al. (25), relatively little similarity is observed in the molecular weights and abundance of the individual polypeptides of HSV-1 and HSV-2.

F.   Enumeration and Differentiation between Structural and Nonstructural Polypeptides in HSV-2 Infected HEp-2 Cells

The mobilities of labeled ICP and VP were compared by simultaneous electrophoresis. Autoradiography of parallel separations indicates that cells infected with HSV-2 (G strain) synthesize 53 polypeptides, whereas under the same conditions, only 24 bands were resolved in separations of proteins from purified virions. These ICP were assigned numbers 1–53 in order of descending molecular

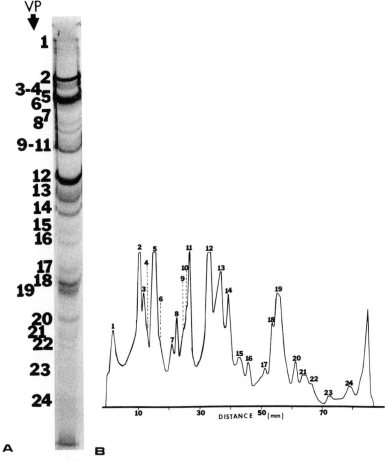

Figure 4. Autoradiograms of electrophoretically separated [³⁵S]methionine-labeled virion polypeptides (purified from cells and labeled 6–24 hr post-infection). Solubilized labeled virions were subjected to electrophoresis in 8.5% gels and processed for autoradiography. *A*, reproduction of photograph of the original autoradiogram; *B*, absorbance profiles of the same autoradiogram. Virus-specific protein bands have been assigned numbers from 1 to 24 (VP 1–VP 24).

weight and independent of the virion protein numbering (i.e., VP 1–24). An ICP with the same electrophoretic mobility as a VP was considered analogous to the VP and designated structural. ICP with electrophoretic mobilities different from those of VP were designated

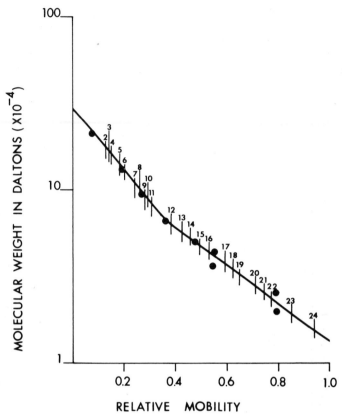

Figure 5. Molecular weights of HSV-2 (G) virion polypeptides determined from their migration relative to protein standards of known molecular weight on 8.5% polyacrylamide gels. The standards are: Myosin (212,000 daltons), β-galactosidase (130,000 daltons), phosphorylase B (92,500 daltons), heavy chain of human IgM (76,000 daltons), Bovine serum albumin (67,000 daltons), ovalbumin (44,500 daltons), light chain of human IgG (20,000 daltons). The position of virion polypeptides is indicated by vertical line intersecting the curve connecting standard proteins and annotated with the appropriate numerical designation. The migrations of standard proteins and of virion polypeptides were calculated as a fraction of the distance migrated by bromphenol blue dye.

nonstructural or host. Criteria accepted as evidence that ICP are virus specified are based on three types of experiments: (a) comparisons of polypeptides synthesized in infected and uninfected cells, (b) specific precipitation by antisera reacting solely with virus-specific antigens, and (c) comparisons of HSV-2 (G) ICP with ICP made in cells infected with other variants of the virus. Similar criteria were accepted by Honess and Roizman for HSV-1 (*25*). Comparison of polypeptides synthesized in cells infected with HSV-2 or mock-infected and labeled with [^{35}S]methionine from 12 to 16 hr after infection indicates that over similar regions, a higher rate of synthesis can be observed in the infected cells (Figure 6).

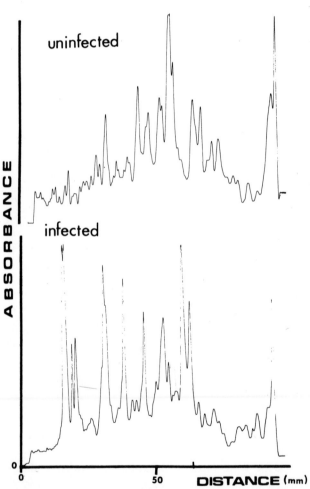

Figure 6. Absorbance profiles of autoradiographic images of electrophoretically separated proteins from infected (*bottom tracing*) and uninfected cells (*top tracing*) labeled 12–16 hr after infection or mock infection. Proteins were separated on 8.5% polyacrylamide gels.

This criterion (induction) was further analyzed in a series of experiments designed to investigate the kinetics of synthesis of individual ICP. Infected cultures were labeled at 0–4, 4–8, 8–12, and 12–16 hr postinfection, respectively. The autoradiograms of the gels were scanned with a Joyce-Loebel Chromoscan equipped with an integrator. The integrator records a number of counts proportional to the product of the horizontal and vertical displacements of the pen. The number of integrator counts under any one peak of the scan was divided by the total number of integrator counts for the entire scan to give the fraction of total radioactivity found in the peak. Analysis of the kinetics of ICP synthesis (Table 4) shows either a gradual increase, or an initial increase followed by a leveling off or a decline in 47 of these ICP. These polypeptides are accepted as virus-specific. Since host protein synthesis is inhibited in HSV infected cells, polypeptides showing a gradual decrease were considered to be of host origin (53). Comparison of the rates of synthesis of the structural polypeptides at various time intervals with the amounts of these polypeptides in the virion, show that they are not synthesized in proportion to their incorporation into virus particle. A pertinent example is a minor virion protein (VP 4), made in large abundance in the infected cell between 4 and 12 hr after infection.

G. Effect of Inhibition of Infected Cell
Protein Synthesis on Subsequent Synthesis of AG-4

HEp-2 cells were infected with 10 PFU of HSV-2 per cell and incubated at 37°C for 8 hr in the presence of 50 μg/ml of cycloheximide. At this time they were overlayed with minimum essential medium (MEM) containing [^{35}S]methionine (10 μCi/ml) and 10 μg/ml of actinomycin D and reincubated for 4, 6, and 8 hr. The rationale for this approach, based on the studies of Honess and Roizman (24) with HSV-1, is 2-fold. First, the HSV-1 polypeptides made immediately upon removal of cycloheximide represent a subset of the ICP made in untreated cells at this time. They correspond to proteins normally made early in infection and do not require prior infected cell protein synthesis in order to be made. Second, actinomycin D prevents or reduces the decline in the rates of synthesis of this subset of proteins, at the same time precluding the synthesis of other sets of viral polypeptides. Complement-fixing activity with AG-4 positive sera is borderline (10% fixation) in HEp-2 cells

Table 4. Enumeration, classification, and evidence for virus specificity of HSV-2 (G) ICP

ICP[a] no.	Classification	M.W. (daltons)	Period of Synthesis (hr p.i.)	Period of Max. Synthesis (hr p.i.)[b]	Precipitated by anti-SAM[c]
1	VP[d] 1	262,000	0–16	0–12	
2	H[e]	235,000	0–16	decreases	
3	NS[f]	230,000	0–16	4–12	
4	NS	222,000	0–16	4–8	
5	H	209,000	0–16	decreases	
6	H	200,000	0–16	decreases	
7	NS	195,000	0–12	4–8	
8	VP 2	175,000	0–16	4–12	+
9	VP 3	165,000	0–16	4–12	+
10	VP 4	161,000	0–16	4–8	
11	NS	153,000	0–4	0–4	
12	VP 5	141,000	0–16	4–8	+
13	H	138,000	0–4	decreases	
14	VP 6	130,000	4–16	4–8	+
15	NS	126,000	0–16	4–8	+
16	VP 7	110,000	4–16	8–16	+
17	NS	105,000	4–16	4–8	+
18	VP 8	102,000	0–16	4–8	+
19	VP 9	92,000	8–16	12–16	+
20	VP 10	89,000	4–16	12–16	+

Table 4. continued

ICP[a] no.	Classification	M.W. (daltons)	Period of Synthesis (hr p.i.)	Period of Max. Synthesis (hr p.i.)[b]	Precipitated by anti-SAM[c]
21	VP 11	85,000	4–16	12–16	+
22	NS	77,000	0–16	12–16	
23	NS	75,000	0–8	4–8	
24	NS	72,000	0–4		
25	NS	67,000	0–16	4–8	+
26	NS	64,000	0–16	4–8	+
27	VP 12	62,000	0–16	4–16	+
28	NS	58,000	8–16	12–16	+
29	VP 13	57,000	0–16	4–8	
30	VP 14	52,000	0–16	4–8	
31	NS	51,000	4–16	12–16	+
32	NS	49,000	0–4	0–4	
33	VP 15	47,000	0–16	0–4	
34	VP 16	44,000	8–16	12–16	+
35	NS	41,500	0–16	0–4	+
36	NS	39,500	4–16	12–16	
37	NS	38,000	4–16	12–16	
38	VP 17	37,000	0–16	4–12	+
39	VP 18	34,500	0–16	4–16	+
40	VP 19	32,500	0–16	4–16	+

continued

Table 4. continued

ICP[a] no.	Classification	M.W. (daltons)	Period of Synthesis (hr p.i.)	Period of Max. Synthesis (hr p.i.)[b]	Precipitated by anti-SAM[c]
41	NS	31,500	0–12	0–4	
42	NS	29,500	0–16	0–4	++
43	VP 20	27,500	0–16	4–12	++
44	H	27,000	0–4	decreases	
45	VP 21	25,500	4–16	8–12	
46	VP 22	24,000	0–16	increases	
47	NS	22,800	0–16	increases	
48	H	21,000	0–16	decreases	
49	VP 23	19,500	4–16	8–12	
50	NS	18,200	4–16	8–16	
51	VP 24	15,500	4–16	12–16	++
52	NS	14,900	0–12	0–4	
53	NS	14,100	8–16	12–16	

[a]Infected cell polypeptide.
[b]Hours after infection.
[c]Rabbit serum against total viral soluble proteins, adsorbed with uninfected HEp-2 cells and sheep red blood cells.
[d]Virion protein.
[e]Host protein.
[f]Nonstructural, virus-specified polypeptide.

infected with HSV-2 and exposed to actinomycin D for 8 hr after cycloheximide removal and relatively high (20–38% fixation) in similarly infected cells exposed to actinomycin D for 4 or 6 hr. Fixation is not observed with AG-4 negative sera (Table 5).

Autoradiograms of the electrophoretically separated polypeptides present in these cells are shown in Figure 7, together with polypeptides labeled in uninfected cells untreated and treated in a similar fashion.

Comparisons of these samples showed that most ICP that are made during the pulse interval after removal of cycloheximide cannot be differentiated from the polypeptides of the similarly treated mock infected cells. The exception are seven ICP unique to the infected cells and respectively designated ICP 6, VP 4, VP 5, ICP 25, ICP 26, VP 12, and VP 14 according to their correspondence in electrophoretic mobility to polypeptides from purified virions (VP) or from untreated infected cells labeled at the same time intervals in the virus growth cycle and simultaneously electrophoresed.

Table 5. Complement fixing ability of various antigenic preparations with AG-4 positive and negative sera

	Percent complement fixation	
Fraction	AG-4 positive serum	AG-4 negative serum
HEp-2/G/4 hr[a]	20	0
HEp-2/G/6 hr	38	0
HEp-2/G/8 hr	10	0
HEp-R/G/6 hr	45	0
HEp-R/GW/6 hr	0	0
0.005 M[b]	0	0
0.04 M	53.3%	0
0.06 M	0	0
0.08 M	0	0
0.1 M	12%	0
0.2 M	0	0
0.4 M	0	0
1.0 M	0	0

[a] HEp-2 or HEp-R cells infected with G or GW virus in presence of cycloheximide were labeled with [^{35}S]methionine in presence of actinomycin D for 4, 6, or 8 hr after cycloheximide removal.

[b] Fractions eluted from a brushite column with increasing molar concentrations of phosphate buffer.

110   Aurelian et al.

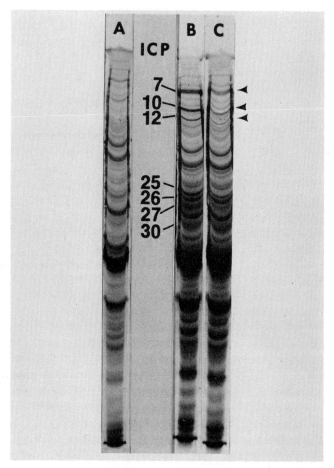

Figure 7. Autoradiograms of 8.5% polyacrylamide gels containing electro-phoretically separated polypeptides from HSV-2 (G) infected HEp-2 cells labeled with [³⁵S]methionine for 4 and 6 hr, starting immediately after removal of cycloheximide added at the time of infection and from cells mock infected, treated with cycloheximide and labeled for the same time interval. Enumeration of ICP identifies those that are virus rather than host specific. Arrows represent the ICP synthesized at higher rates after removal of cycloheximide.

Of major significance is the observation that, although the relative abundance of six of the seven ICPs unique to the infected cells is similar in preparations labeled for 4, 6, and 8 hr after removal of cycloheximide, VP 4 is made in largest amounts in cells exposed to actinomycin D for 4 and 6 hr. In view of the border-line (10%) complement-fixing AG-4 activity of the extracts from the cells exposed to actinomycin D for 8 hr after removal of cyclo-heximide, the data suggest that complement-fixing ability with AG-4 positive, cervical cancer sera, may be associated with the virion polypeptide designated VP 4. The observation that treatment of uninfected cells with cycloheximide does not have a marked selective effect on the polypeptides made after drug removal is expected (24). However, the presence of host polypeptides in the infected cells treated with cycloheximide possibly is more difficult to interpret with currently available data.

H.   Effect of Virus Passage History on
Synthesis of VP 4 in Presence of Cycloheximide

In view of a possible association between VP 4 and AG-4 comple-ment-fixing activity, experiments similar to those described above were performed. Two lines of HEp-2 cells were used: (a) "HEp-2" originally obtained from Microbiological Associates (Bethesda, Maryland) and maintained in our laboratory in medium 199 with 10% calf serum, and (b) "HEp-R," morphologically more fibro-blastic-like than the HEp-2 cells, originally obtained from Dr. B. Roizman (University of Chicago, Chicago, Illinois), and grown in MEM, supplemented with 10% fetal calf serum. Both lines were transferred with EDTA. The HSV-2 stocks used were "G," a virus generally used in AG-4 preparation originally obtained from Dr. Roizman and passaged 60 times in our laboratory in HEp-2 cells at a high multiplicity of infection, and "GW," a low passage seed of G virus further passaged only three times in our laboratory in HEp-R cells at a low multiplicity of infection.

Cells were infected with virus in the presence of 50 μg/ml of cycloheximide. After 8 hr, the drug was removed and the infected cells were exposed to [^{35}S]methionine for 6 hr in the presence of actinomycin D. Extracts from these cells were assayed for their ability to fix complement with AG-4 positive sera. Good fixation (38–45%) was observed in HEp-2 and HEp-R cells infected with G virus, whereas extracts from GW infected HEp-R cells did not fix complement with AG-4 positive sera (Table 5). The following points were made evident by the analysis of the labeled polypeptides separated by polyacrylamide gel electrophoresis (Figure 8).

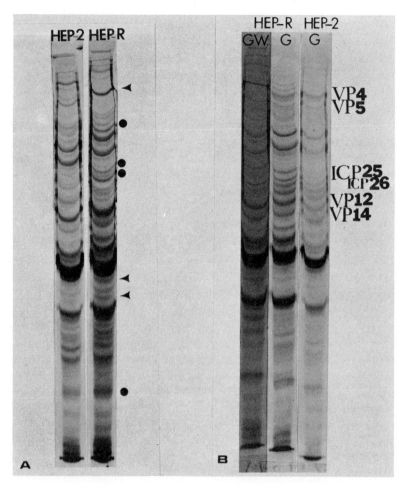

Figure 8. *A*, autoradiograms of polyacrylamide gels containing electrophoretically separated polypeptides from mock infected HEp-2 and HEp-R cells labeled with [^{35}S]methionine for 6 hr starting immediately after removal of cycloheximide added at the time of infection, represent differences in the protein profiles of the two cell clones. *B*, autoradiograms of polyacrylamide gels containing electrophoretically separated polypeptides from HSV-2 (G and GW) infected HEp-2 and HEp-R cells labeled with [^{35}S]methionine for 6 hr starting immediately after removal of cycloheximide added at the time of infection.

(1.) The morphologic differences between HEp-2 and HEp-R cells are reflected in differences in the species and abundance of their polypeptides.

(2.) The polypeptides made in HEp-R cells infected with G virus after removal of cycloheximide are host polypeptides similar to those made in uninfected cells and the same seven ICP that are also present in HEp-2 cells infected with G virus. The relative abundance of these ICP is also similar to that observed in HEp-2 cells infected with G virus.

(3.) One ICP (VP 4) present in both HEp-2 and HEp-R cells infected with G virus is not made in HEp-R cells infected with GW and labeled with [^{35}S]methionine for 6 hr in presence of actinomycin D after removal of cycloheximide. Another ICP (VP 5) is made, although in much lower amounts than in HEp-2 and HEp-R cells infected with G virus under similar conditions. These observations confirm the association between VP 4 and the ability of infected cell extracts to fix complement with AG-4 positive sera. They further indicate that this is a virus-specific function. Studies designed to investigate the association of VP 4 with defective viral DNA are now in progress.

I.   Immunoprecipitation of ^{35}S-Labeled AG-4

Of the polypeptides present in the antigens (Figure 9), only some are precipitated efficiently and some are not precipitated at all by different immune sera. Thus serum No. 12 but not sera No. 9 and 15 precipitate VP 5. All sera precipitate VP 12 and both sera No. 9 and 12 precipitate ICP 26; however, this is also precipitated by the rabbit anti-SAM serum. Finally serum No. 15 and the rabbit anti-SAM serum precipitate VP 14; it is not precipitated by sera No. 9 and 12. Of major significance is the observation that the major polypeptide precipitated by both of the AG-4 positive sera (No. 12 and 9), but not by the AG-4 negative serum (No. 15), is VP 4.

J.   Purification of ^{35}S-Labeled AG-4

Chromatography on Sephadex G-200 followed by calcium phosphate (brushite), prepared according to the method of Taverne (50) was used. AG-4 was made in HEp-2 cells infected with G virus as previously described (2, 3). Eluates were assayed for complement fixing activity with AG-4 positive and negative sera. The elution profile from Sephadex G-200 of the antigen fixing complement with AG-4 positive but not negative sera is shown in Figure 10A. The AG-4 positive fractions were pooled, dialyzed overnight against 0.005 M phosphate buffer (pH 7.0), and chromatographed on

114   Aurelian et al.

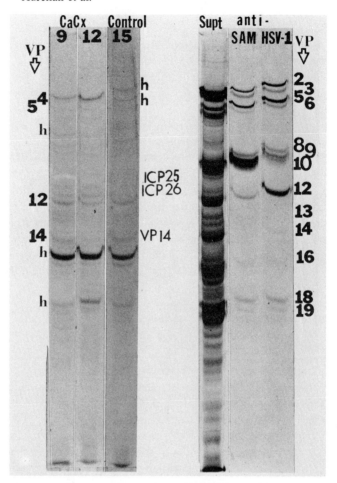

Figure 9. Autoradiograms of 8.5% polyacrylamide gels containing electro-phoretically separated immune precipitates formed by the addition of AG-4 positive (Nos. 12 and 9) or AG-4 negative (No. 15) sera to supernatant fluid from high-speed centrifugation of infected cells lysate labeled with [³⁵S]methio-nine for 6 hr, starting immediately after removal of cycloheximide. Immune precipitates formed by the addition of antiserum specific for soluble HSV-2 (G) proteins (anti-SAM) or HSV-1 (anti-HSV-1). Numbers on the sides refer to virus-specific ICP precipitated by the various antisera.

calcium phosphate. Figure 10*B* shows the elution profile of the proteins removed from the column in a stepwise fashion with increasing concentrations of phosphate buffer. Eluates were dialyzed against veronal buffer, assayed for complement fixing activity with AG-4

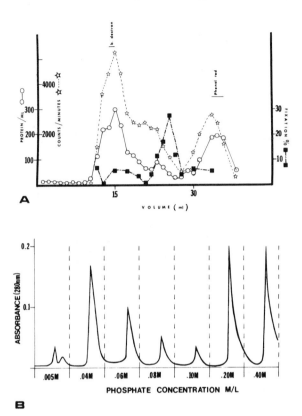

Figure 10. *A*, elution profile of proteins removed from a Sephadex G-200 column represent complement fixing activity with AG-4 positive sera; *B*, elution profile of proteins removed from a brushite column in a stepwise fashion with increasing concentrations of potassium phosphate buffer pH 7.0 containing 0.1 M NaCl. For this experiment Sephadex G-200 fractions fixing complement with AG-4 positive sera were pooled, and applied to the column in 0.005 M phosphate buffer.

positive and negative sera, solubilized, and electrophoresed on polyacrylamide gels. Two fractions, one eluted with 0.04 M and the other with 0.1 M phosphate buffer, fixed complement with AG-4 positive but not with AG-4 negative sera (Table 5). AG-4 reactivity was not observed in any other fraction. The major complement fixing activity (53% fixation) resides in the fraction eluted with 0.04 M buffer, whereas only 12% fixation is obtained with the fraction eluted with 0.1 M buffer. Autoradiograms of the polyacrylamide gels of these fractions (Figure 11) indicate the 0.04 M eluate contains

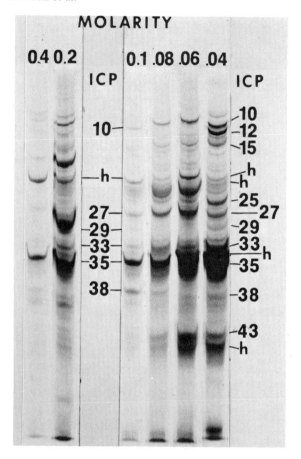

Figure 11. Autoradiograms of 8.5% polyacrylamide gels containing electrophoretically separated polypeptides from fractions eluted from a brushite column with increasing concentrations of potassium phosphate buffer pH 7.0 containing 0.1 M NaCl.

13 major polypeptides including VP 4 and VP 5, whereas only 6 major polypeptides are observed in the 0.1 M calcium phosphate fraction. The only polypeptide unique to both these fractions and absent from all others is VP 4. Furthermore, its relative abundance in the two fractions corresponds to their complement-fixing ability, being much higher in the 0.04 M than the 0.1 M eluate.

The studies described in these sections associate AG-4 complement-fixing activity with VP 4, a minor virion protein of 161,000 daltons. The presence of AG-4 on the surface of infected cells does not negate the interpretation since (a) all virus-specific proteins binding to membranes are also structural proteins of the virus, (b) not all surface HSV-1 antigens are glycosylated, and (c) in the virion, the virus specific glycoproteins are structural components of the envelope usually derived from the inner lamella of the nuclear membrane (20). On the other hand, the data do not allow differentiation between two possibilities pertaining to the location of AG-4 in the virion. Thus it is possible that AG-4 is a subsurface virion protein. Alternatively, AG-4 is located on the virion surface but is too minor a protein to be of quantitative significance in virus neutralization. The latter is not a very probable interpretation because extracts of infected cells used in the blocking experiments contained VP 4 in relatively high abundance (Table 4).

III. CELL-MEDIATED IMMUNITY TO HERPESVIRUS

It has become evident that immune responses, humoral and/or cellular, play a significant role in herpesvirus infections. Thus, Stevens and Cook (49) have shown that IgG in latently infected mice prevents total viral reactivation in transplanted syngeneic latently infected ganglia. However, others suggest that both the humoral and the cellular immune (CMI) systems must operate together in a synergistic fashion to suppress herpesvirus infections (33). Indeed, the data of Wilton et al. indicate that predisposition to recurrent lesions is a function of the absence of macrophage-migration inhibition factor (MIF) and lymphocyte cytotoxin (52). Immunosuppressive therapy and syndromes associated with alteration of the humoral and cell-mediated immune systems increase the number and/or severity of lesions due to herpesvirus recurrences, and, finally, lymphocytes independently or in concert with macrophages may produce interferon resulting in reduced or limited viral replication in neighboring uninfected cells (19, 42). The mechanism and the regulation of CMI responses to the herpesviruses, the specific virus polypeptides that are immunogenic, modulating humoral and/ or cellular responses, and the relationship of both these factors to disease (productive, latent, and cancer) constitute the focus of many present investigations.

The experiments described below were designed to examine some of these points.

A. Cell-mediated Immunity in Primary Herpesvirus Infections

Primary exposure to HSV-1 occurs generally early in life in approximately 85% of people (28); primary infection with HSV-2 follows puberty (36) and occurs mostly in people with a previous HSV-1 infection, i.e., in presence of highly cross-reacting neutralizing antibody. This observation gives rise to three questions. First, does infection with HSV-2 occur in presence of high levels of neutralizing antibody because of a deficient CMI response? Second, what is the in vivo interaction between humoral and cell-mediated responses, and how are they regulated? The ability of antibody to potentiate or inhibit CMI responses in vitro has been described (26). Finally the question arises as to the validity of various in vitro assays for the understanding of in vivo CMI responses, in general, and to herpesvirus antigens in particular.

Rabbits were infected with 2×10^7 PFU of HSV-1 (F strain) or HSV-2 (G strain) by foot pad inoculation and their ability to respond to viral antigens by lymphocyte blastogenesis was determined at 0, 4, 7, 10, 15, and 22 days after infection. This assay was selected because it had been shown to have a broad spectrum, capable of identifying the responses of both memory and effector cell subpopulations (23). However, it should be stressed that the ability of the various in vitro assays to assess CMI is not completely understood. Available evidence suggests they correlate with delayed hypersensitivity (8, 38).

Briefly, peripheral blood leukocytes (PBL) were obtained from freshly drawn heparinized blood, allowed to settle for 30 min at 37°C in the presence of 0.2% Methocel (15 cps). Cells from poplietal lymph nodes and spleens were obtained by filtration through 200-mesh stainless steel screens. Following centrifugation, cells were resuspended in medium RPMI 1640 (Grand Island Biological), supplemented with 5% heat-inactivated fetal calf serum, and centrifuged at $400 \times g$ for 20 min at ambient temperature, on a Ficoll-Hypaque gradient (70 ml of 9% Ficoll 400, Pharmacia Piscataway, New Jersey, and 30 ml of 32.8% w/v sodium metrizoate solution, Gallard-Schlesinger Chemical Co, Carle Place, New York). The cells at the interface were aspirated, washed in Hanks' Balanced Salt Solution (BSS), and exposed to 0.83% ammonium chloride (in H_2O) to lyse any remaining red blood cells. Following two more cycles of washing in RPMI 1640, cells were counted and viability determined by trypan blue exclusion. Routine yields consisted of 98% mononuclear cells and 60–80% recovery. Cultures (0.2 ml) were set in flat-bottom Limbro microtiter plates containing 1–2×10^6 viable cells/ml and 25 μl of the appropriate antigen, i.e., (a) HSV-1 (F strain) and HSV-2 (G strain) purified of soluble proteins by centrifugation at 25,000 rpm for 1.5 hr in a Spinco SW 27 rotor, and (b) AG-4 and AG-H prepared as described (1, 2). Following incubation in a 5% CO_2 atmosphere at 37°C for 72 hr, cultures were pulsed for 4 hr with μCi of [^{3}H]thymidine (New England Nuclear, specific activity 55.3 Ci/mM), and harvested with a multiple automatic sample harvester (MASH, Biotechnology Inst.). MASH collects the contents of 12 cells simultaneously, washes them individually, filters the fluids from each well, and eliminates the unbound label from the filters. Following harvesting, the filter strips were dried and the individual filter spots torn from the strip along the old ring impression and counted with Bray's solution in a Packard scintillation counter. The advantages of the microtest assay are that it (a) allows for more tests per sample, (b) requires little incubation space, (c) allows for testing of small volumes and accordingly of increasing antigen concentrations, (d) is easy to perform, and (e) causes a sharp decrease in error between replicate samples, giving rise to high reproducibility (54). Furthermore, in simultaneous assays in our laboratory, comparison of this microtest to the usually employed tube macrotest procedure (45) indicates the microtest is at least 3- to 5-fold more sensitive and of similar specificity.

The results of the lymphocyte blastogenesis assay are expressed as stimulation indices (SI) and represent:

$$\frac{\text{stimulation in presence of antigen}}{\text{stimulation in presence of control medium}}$$

Three questions were asked in the studies described in this and the following sections. First, what are the kinetics and the magnitude of primary blastogenic responses to the herpesvirus antigens and are they specific to the infecting virus type? Second, does first infection with either virus type (HSV-1 or HSV-2) affect the blastogenic response to the other one? Third, does circulating antibody affect the blastogenic response to either virus type? Blastogenic responses to HSV-1 and HSV-2 first observed at 4 days were maximal at 10 days after infection. Positive responses were still observed 12 days later (Figure 12). The magnitude of the response (Table 6) appeared to reflect a gradient of antigen processing. Thus, best responses (SI = 50) were observed in cultures of poplietal lymph nodes draining the site of infection. The responses were weaker in spleen cultures (SI = 15) and weakest (SI = 7) in peripheral blood cultures. In complete agreement with the close antigenic similarity of HSV-1 and HSV-2, animals exposed to either virus type respond to both viruses (*31, 36*). However, the magnitude of the response is higher for the homologous virus, as previously reported by Rosenberg et al. (*46*). Virus specificity can therefore be expressed as a ratio of the stimulation index for HSV-1 to that for HSV-2 at a specific antigen concentration. Under these conditions a ratio of 1 or higher is obtained in cell cultures from animals exposed to HSV-1, whereas a ratio lower than 1 represents the response of cell cultures from animals exposed to HSV-2.

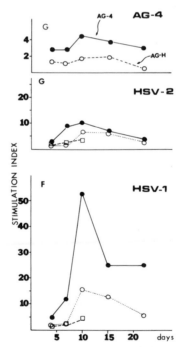

Figure 12. Kinetics of blastogenic response to HSV-1, HSV-2, and AG-4 in rabbits following primary infection with HSV-1 (F) or HSV-2 (G). Response to AG-4 is plotted only for animals infected with HSV-2. HSV-1 immune animals do not respond to AG-4. Lymph node cultures, ● — ●; spleen cultures, ○ .... ○; and PBL cultures, □ - - - □.

Table 6. In vitro stimulation of immune lymphocytes from PBL, lymph nodes, and spleen with HSV-1 and HSV-2

[³H]Thymidine Uptake

Antigen	Spleen cultures from rabbits with primary		Lymph node cultures from rabbits with primary		PBL cultures from rabbits with primary		Lymph node cultures from HSV-1 hyperimmune rabbits challenged with	
	HSV-1	HSV-2	HSV-1	HSV-2	HSV-1	HSV-2	HSV-1	HSV-2
HSV-1	38,274	8,987	28,963	67,298	1,730	2,113	34,892	13,830
HSV-2	20,105	20,007	17,390	168,892	1,282	3,664	18,274	15,907
PBS	2,802	1,783	3,599	6,481	758	445	12,223	11,562
ConA	120,609	164,136	143,960	239,760	9,096	4,460	218,838	245,673

Significantly, AG-4 specific in vitro stimulation of lymph node cultures was observed as early as 4 days after primary exposure of the animals to HSV-2, with peak responses being evident at 10 days postinfection (Figure 12). Antibody to AG-4 was not present at this time. AG-4 specific blastogenesis was not observed in animals with primary HSV-1 infections, and in animals hyperimmunized with either virus type. This observation, as well as the inability of animals with a primary HSV-2 infection to recognize another viral antigen designated CP-1 (10), suggests that AG-4 is immunogenic and can induce CMI-related responses independently of the virion itself. It is not clear at present whether blastogenesis signifies the initial events of antibody synthesis, or those of cell-mediated immunity, or both (38).

The ability to mount a blastogenic response to AG-4 following primary infection with HSV-2 suggests that women with cervical cancer must possess memory cells capable of recognizing this antigen. The significance of this interpretation rests on the recognition that AG-4 is a virion protein present only in tissues from cervical cancer and is associated with the active tumor growth.

B. Cell-mediated Immunity in Latency

Following recovery from the primary infection, a fraction of the population suffers from recurrent lesions appearing at or near the site of the primary infection. Recurrent lesions can be predicted and are induced by a variety of stress provocations such as sun, strong wind, fever, hormone therapy, menstruation, etc. (44). The predictable character of recurrences and their occurrence always at the same site on the body suggests that they are not due to reinfection, but rather are derived from an endogenous virus residing in the body in the interim between recrudescences. These conclusions are corroborated by the observation that people suffering from recurrences have high levels of circulating neutralizing antibody. Nevertheless, exogenous reinfection has been described and is most obvious in the case of infection with HSV-2, which occurs at puberty in presence of antibody to HSV-1 (36).

Two questions were asked in the studies described in this section. First, whether blastogenic responses of hyperimmune animals are similar to those in animals with primary infections, and second, whether immune surveillance plays a role in the maintenance of latency. In order to examine the effect of prior exposure to herpesvirus on the ability of the host to develop cellular reactivity against a new incoming herpesvirus, animals were hyperimmunized with either of the virus types and rechallenged with HSV-1 or HSV-2. Their blastogenic response to HSV-1 and HSV-2 was studied at 4, 7, 10, and 15 days after the challenge. The results of these studies may be summarized as follows:

1. Animals infected simultaneously with HSV-1 in the left foot pad and HSV-2 in the right foot pad respond equally well to both virus types. Poplietal lymph node cultures display virus specificity with cells from the left lymph node reacting as HSV-1 specific, and those from the right one as HSV-2 specific. On the other hand, spleen cultures from those animals recognize only HSV-1.

2. Animals hyperimmunized with HSV-1 and challenged with the homologous virus display antigen-specific blastogenesis to HSV-1. The magnitude of the response is at least 2-fold lower than the one detected following primary HSV-1 infection. HSV-1 hyperimmune animals challenged with HSV-2 do not respond to HSV-2, but remain positive for HSV-1 (Table 6).

3. Antibody to either or both virus types can enhance or decrease the blastogenic response.

The data indicate that infection with either virus type has an inhibitory effect on the host's ability to mount a blastogenic response toward a superinfecting virus. This is particularly evident when, as in humans, the host is HSV-1 immune and HSV-2 is the challenging virus. The exact role of circulating antibody in the mechanisms of such phenomena is now under investigation in our laboratory.

The involvement of cellular reactivity to the herpesviruses in the maintenance of the state of latency was monitored in people with a history of recurrent herpetic infections. Blood samples were collected prior to recurrence, at the peak of recurrence, and 10–15 days after resolution of the lesions. Two in vitro assays were used, the lymphocyte blastogenesis and the leukocyte migration inhibition. The latter assay was selected since it has been shown to be ideal for the study of CMI to latent infections in immunologically compromised patients and displays complete correlation with the results of skin tests for delayed hypersensitivity (16). In this assay, polymorphonuclear (PMN) pellets obtained following Ficoll-Hypaque gradients were washed with BSS, counted, and mixed at a 1:1 ratio with the mononuclear cells. Final concentrations consisted of 1.5 $\times$

10^8 viable cells/ml in medium 199 containing 10% horse serum and the appropriate antigen. The cell suspension was incubated 30 min at $37°C$ and placed ($10 \ \mu l$/well) in wells (2.5 mm in diameter) punched in a plate of 0.65% Special Noble Agar (Difco) in medium 199 (GIBCO) with 10% horse serum. Following 22 hr incubation at $37°C$ in a 5% CO_2 atmosphere, the cells were fixed by exposure to 10% acetic acid for an additional 48 hr and stained with 0.25% Ponceau-S in 3% trichloroacetic acid for an additional 48 hr. Since cell migration occurs on the surface of the plates, the agar overlay was gently removed and areas of migration measured at low-power magnification. The results of these assays are expressed as migration inhibition indices (MI) and represent

$$\frac{\text{mean area of migration in medium containing antigen}}{\text{mean area of migration in medium control}}$$

Although preliminary, the results of this study (Figure 13) indicate that in individuals studied at the peak of recurrence, migration is not inhibited by either virus type; virus-specific inhibition is observed 15 days after resolution of the lesion. Significantly, when a new recurrence is observed, the ability to inhibit migration is abruptly lost. Although decreased in magnitude, antigen-specific blastogenesis is still observed in individuals studied at the peak of recurrence. The data suggest that a defect in immune surveillance is associated with recurrent disease. They do not prove causation nor do they exclude the possible involvement of the humoral response in maintaining a state of latency (49). Of particular interest is the observation that individuals with recurrent HSV-2 infections do not respond to AG-4 by either one of the in vitro assays used in these studies. In view of the detection of AG-4 specific blastogenesis in animals with primary but not hyperimmune HSV-2 infections, this lack of response is amenable to three interpretations: (a) CMI responses are of relatively short duration and require the continuous presence of circulating antigen. Following primary infection, the amount of circulating AG-4 is too low for recognition. (b) The level of AG-4 in circulation is relatively high; however, hyperimmune individuals are immunologically impaired. This is not very probable because such individuals can mount cellular reactivity to the virions. (c) CMI responses to AG-4 are inhibited by circulating AG-4 antibody or antigen-antibody complexes.

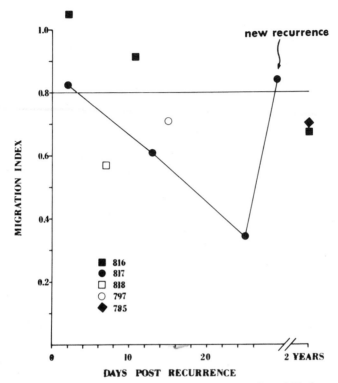

Figure 13. Leukocyte migration inhibition (MI lower than 0.8) in patients with recurrent herpetic lesions. Recurrence is associated with loss of migration inhibition. Numbers represent various individuals studied.

C. Cell-mediated Immunity to HSV-2
Antigens in Patients with Cervical Cancer and Controls

The observation that patients with cervical cancer are not anergic suggests that some HSV antigens should be recognized by the host, and they should show response in CMI assays. Three hypotheses could explain the possible involvement of the cellular response to viral antigens in cervical cancer.

1. The development of cervical neoplasia may be the result of an alteration of the immunologic surveillance system, manifested specifically by an impaired ability to recognize and/or eliminate tumor cells displaying a tumor-specific, virus-coded antigen. It would then follow that women who are seropositive for HSV-2

and fail to develop cervical cancer but develop atypia do not exhibit a similar immunologic impairment.

2. The development of cervical cancer is accompanied by the appearance on tumor cells of a tumor-specific, virus-coded antigen, which in turn stimulates clones of antigen reactive lymphocytes. Implicit in this hypothesis is that lymphocytes from HSV-2 seropositive individuals without evidence of cervical neoplasia would react either minimally or not at all to these antigens.

3. There is neither an impaired nor an enhanced immunologic reactivity at the effector lymphocyte level. However, tumor induction is accompanied by the development of specific antibody populations that can act as "blocking" antibody either by binding to antigen recognition sites, or to the tumor-specific, virus-coded antigen on the tumor cells, rendering them inaccessible to effector lymphocytes. It should be pointed out that VP 4 is a good candidate for the role of the tumor-specific virus-coded antigen essential in all three hypotheses, as it fulfills all required criteria.

Preliminary studies designed to inquire into the blastogenic response of patients with cervical cancer and controls (Table 7) may be summarized as follows: (a) the frequency of HSV-2 induced blastogenesis is similar in patients with invasive cancer, preinvasive cancer and controls, and correlates with the frequency of antibody to HSV-2. Accordingly, cellular reactivity to the virus cannot be associated with development of cervical neoplasia. (b) Comparisons of the HSV-2 and HSV-1 induced blastogenesis in cancer and control groups indicate that cancer groups preferentially recognize HSV-2, whereas controls preferentially recognize HSV-1. These results correlate with the previous observation that women with cervical cancer have a higher prevalence of antibody to HSV-2 than control women. (c) AG-4 specific blastogenesis is not observed in control women nor in women with invasive cancers, treated or recurrent. It is observed in 2/12 (17%) preinvasive cancers (atypia and carcinoma in situ). Significantly, the two positive atypia cases and all the untreated or recurrent invasive cancers are AG-4 seropositive. AG-4 seronegative preinvasive cases are nonresponders in blastogenesis assays.

The data indicate that VP 4 is associated with impaired blastogenic responses in patients with invasive cervical cancer. These results are not due to the foreign nature of AG-4 because these women are HSV-2 and AG-4 seropositive. Of particular significance

Table 7. Humoral and cellular reactivity to herpesvirus antigens in patients with cervical cancer and controls

Patient no.	Stimulation index			Antibody to	
	HSV-1	HSV-2	AG-4	HSV-2	AG-4
Atypia					
698	1.2	2.1	< 1	+	−
704	3.2	2.9	4.4	+	+
705	7.8	12.6	< 1	+	−
706	1.7	2.4	< 1	+	−
707	< 1	3.9	< 1	+	−
715	< 1	3.4	< 1	+	−
726	4.9	1.5	< 1	−	−
748	2.3	2.1	< 1	+	−
754	< 1	< 1	< 1	+	−
766	2.2	1.0	< 1	ND	−
In situ					
697	2.9	4.0	ND	+	+
708	1.1	< 1	< 1	+	−
744	2.8	5.2	2.0	+	+
Invasive					
700	4.4	1.1	< 1	+	+
714	< 1	3.0	< 1	+	−
718 treated	9.0	7.8	< 1	+	−
745 treated	2.0	1.9	< 1	+	−
696	1.3	8.5	< 1	+	+
771	1.6	1.3	< 1	+	+
788	3.7	2.1	< 1	+	+
Controls					
757	2.3	1.7	1.4	−	−
755	4.0	2.1	< 1	−	−
663	3.8	1.5	< 1	−	−
701	4.4	2.8	< 1	−	−
684	1.0	1.5	< 1	+	−
702	5.0	3.7	< 1	+	−
720	7.1	1.8	< 1	+	−
703	< 1	3.3	< 1	−	−
732	1.2	1.4	< 1	−	−
756	< 1	< 1	< 1	+	−
762	2.1	1.4	< 1	−	−
760	1.3	1.7	< 1	−	−

in view of the hypotheses describing the possible involvement of cellular responses to herpesvirus antigens in cervical cancer is the observation that women with precancerous lesions do not exhibit a similar impairment.

ACKNOWLEDGMENTS

We wish to express our gratitude to Dr. G. Cole and Dr. R. L. Marcus for invaluable help and criticism, to Dr. H. J. Davis and Dr. N. B. Rosenshein for clinical support, to Mrs. R. Miante, Miss M. Albuerne, and Miss L. Sachs for excellent technical assistance, and Miss B. Hurtt for help with the manuscript.

LITERATURE CITED

1. Anzai, T., G. R. Dreasman, R. J. Courtney, E. Adam, W. E. Rawls, and M. Beryesh-Melnick (1975). Antibody to herpes simplex virus type 2 induced nonstructural proteins in women with cervical cancer and control groups. J. Nat. Cancer Inst. 54:1051–1059.

2. Aurelian, L., H. J. Davis, and C. G. Julian (1973). Herpesvirus type 2 induced tumor specific antigen in cervical carcinoma. Am. J. Epid. 98:1–9.

3. Aurelian, L., B. Schumann, and R. L. Marcus (1973). Antibody to HSV-2 induced tumor specific antigens in sera from patients with cervical carcinoma. Science 181:161–164.

4. Aurelian, L., I. Royston, and H. J. Davis (1970). Antibody to genital herpesvirus: Association with cervical atypia and carcinoma in situ. J. Nat. Cancer Inst. 45:455–464.

5. Aurelian, L., J. D. Strandberg, and H. J. Davis (1972). HSV-2 antigens absent from biopsied cervical tumor cells: A model consistent with latency. Proc. Soc. Exp. Biol. Med. 140:404–408.

6. Aurelian, L., J. D. Strandberg, L. V. Melendez, and L. A. Johnson (1968). Herpesvirus type 2 isolated from cervical cells grown in tissue culture. Science 174:485–488.

7. Aurelian, L., J. D. Cornish, and M. F. Smith (1975). Herpesvirus type II-induced tumor specific antigen (AG-4) and specific antibody in patients with cervical cancer and controls. Oncogenesis and Herpesviruses II. p. 79–87.

8. Bennett, B. and B. R. Bloom (1968). Reactions in vivo and in vitro produced by a soluble substance associated with delayed type hypersensitivity. Proc. Nat. Acad. Sci. U.S.A. 59:756–762.

9. Bronson, D. L., G. R. Dreasman, N. Biswel, and M. Beryesh-Melnick (1973). Defective virions of herpes simplex viruses. Intervirology 1:141–153.

10. Cohen, G. H., M. P. Ponce DeLeon, and C. Nichols (1972). Isolation of a herpes simplex virus-specific antigenic fraction which stimulates the production of neutralizing antibody. J. Virol. 10:1021–1030.

11. Collard, W., H. Thornton, and M. Green (1973). Cells transformed by human herpesvirus type 2 transcribe virus specific RNA se-

quences shared by herpesvirus types 1 and 2. Nature New Biol. 243:264–266.

12. Dimmock, N. J. and D. H. Watson (1969). Proteins specified by influenza virus in infected cells: Analysis by polyacrylamide gel electrophoresis of antigen not present in the virus particles. J. Gen. Virol. 5:499–509.

13. Darai, G. and K. Munk (1973). Human embryonic cancer cells abortively infected with herpesvirus hominis type 2 show some properties of cell transformation. Nature 241:268–269.

14. Fairbanks, G., T. L. Stock, and D. F. H. Wallach (1971). Electrophoretic analysis of the major polypeptides of the human erythrocyte membrane. Biochemistry 10:2606–2617.

15. Frenkel, N., B. Roizman, E. Cassai, and A. J. Nahmias (1972). A DNA fragment of herpes simplex 2 and its transcripts in human cervical cancer tissue. Proc. Nat. Acad. Sci. U.S.A. 69:3784–3789.

16. Gaines, J. D., F. G. Araujo, J. L. Krahenbuhl, and J. S. Remington: Simplified in vitro method for measuring delayed hypersensitivity to latent intracellular infection in Man (Toxoplasmosis). J. Immunol. 109:179–182.

17. Gall, S. A. and H. Haines (1974). Cervical cancer antigens (CCA) and their relationship to herpesvirus. V. Abstract 5th Ann. Meeting Soc. Gynec. Oncologists. Key Biscayne, Florida, January 1974.

18. Garfinkle, B. and B. R. McAuslan (1974). Transformation of cultured mammalian cells by viable herpes simplex virus subtype 1 and 2. Proc. Nat. Acad. Sci. U.S.A. 71:220–224.

19. Glasgow, L. A. (1970). Cellular immunity in host resistance to viral infections. Arch. Int. Med. 126:125–134.

20. Heine, J .W., P. G. Spear, and B. Roizman (1972). Proteins sepcified by herpes simplex virus. VI. Viral Proteins in the plasma membrane. J. Virol. 9:431–439.

21. Hollinshead, A. C., O. Lee, P. B. Chretian, J. L. Tarpley, W. E. Rawls, and E. Adam (1973). Antibodies to herpesvirus nonvirion antigens in squamous carcinomas. Science 182:713–715.

22. Herrera, L., L. Valenciano, F. Sanchez-Garrido, and J. Botella-Llusia (1974). On findings of virus-like structures in uterine cervical carcinoma. Acta Cytol. 18:45–50.

23. Hollander, N., H. Ginsburg, and M. Feedman (1974). In vitro generation of memory lymphocytes reactive to transplantation antigens. J. Exp. Med. 140:1057–1067.

24. Honess, R. W. and B. Roizman (1974). Regulation of herpesvirus macromolecular synthesis. J. Virol. 14:8–19.

25. Honess, R. W. and B. Roizman (1973). Proteins specified by herpes simplex virus. XI. Identification and relative molar rates of synthesis of structural and nonstructural herpes virus polypeptides in the infected cell. J. Virol. 12:1347–1365.

26. Jacobs, R. P., R. M. Blaese, and J. J. Oppenheim (1972). Inhibition of antigen-stimulated in vitro proliferation of thymic dependent

chicken spleen cells by specific antibody. J. Immunol. 109:324–333.

27. Jones, H. W., Jr., K. P. Katayama, A. Stafl, and H. J. Davis (1967). Chromosomes of cervical atypia, carcinoma in situ and epidermoid carcinoma of the cervix. Obst. Gynec. 30:790.

28. Kaplan, A. S. (1969). Herpes Simplex and Pseudorabies Viruses. Springer-Verlag, New York.

29. Kessler, I. I. (1974). Perspectives in the epidemiology of cervical cancer with special reference to the herpesvirus hypothesis. Cancer Res. 34:1091–1110.

30. Kessler, I. I. and L. Aurelian (1975). In: Uterine Cervix in Cancer Epidemiology and Prevention, D. Schottenfeld, Ed., pp. 263-317. Charles C. Thomas, New York.

31. Kieff, E., B. Hoyer, S. L. Bachenheimer, and B. Roizman (1972). Genetic relatedness of type 1 and type 2 herpes simplex viruses. J. Virol. 9:738–745.

32. Koss, L. G. (1969). Concept of genesis and development of carcinoma of the cervix. Obst. Gynec. Survey 24:850–860.

33. Lodmell, D. A., A. Niwa, K. Hayashi, and A. L. Notkins (1973). Prevention of cell-to-cell spread of herpes simplex virus by leukocytes. J. Exp. Med. 137: 706–720.

34. Melvin, P. and L. S. Kucera (1975). Induction of human cell DNA synthesis by herpes simplex virus type 2. J. Virol. 15:534–539.

35. McDevitt, H. O. and M. Landy (1972). Genetic control of immune responsiveness: Relationship to disease susceptibility. Proc. of Int. Conf. Brook Lodge, Augusta, Michigan. Academic Press, New York.

36. Nahmias, A. J. and B. Roizman (1973). Infection with herpes simplex virus 1 and 2. N. Engl. J. Med. 289:667–674.

37. Naib, M., A. J. Nahmias, W. E. Josey, and J. H. Kramer (1964). Genital herpetic infection: Association with cervical dysplasia and carcinoma. Cancer 23:940–945.

38. Oppenheim, J. J. (1968). Relationship of in vitro lymphocyte transformation to delayed hypersensitivity in guinea pigs and man. Fed. Proc. 27:21–28.

39. Palmer, A. E., W. T. London, A. J. Nahmias, Z. M. Naib, Y. Tuncs, D. A. Fucilla, J. H. Ellenberg, and J. L. Cerer (1976). A preliminary report on investigation of oncogenic potential of Herpes simplex virus type 2 in cebus monkeys. Cancer Res. 36:807–809.

40. Rapp, F. and R. Duff (1973). Transformation of hamster embryo fibroblasts by herpes simplex viruses type 1 and type 2. Cancer Res. 33:1524–1534.

41. Rapp, F., R. Conner, R. Glaser, and R. Duff (1972). Absence of Leukosis virus markers in hamster cells transformed by herpes simplex virus type 2. J. Virol. 9:1059–1063.

42. Rasmussen, L. E., G. W. Jordan, D. A. Stevens, and T. C. Merigan (1974). Lymphocyte interferon production and transformation

after herpes simplex infections in humans. J. Immunol. 112:728–736.
43. Reedman, B. M. and G. Klein (1973). Cellular localization of an Epstein-Barr virus (EBV) associated complement-fixing antigen in producer and nonproducer lymphoblastoid cell lines. Int. J. Cancer 11:499.
44. Roizman, B. (1965). An inquiry into the mechanism of recurrent herpes infections of man. In: Perspectives in Virology IV, M. Pollard, Ed., pp. 283–304. Harper and Row, New York.
45. Rosenberg, G. L., P. A. Farber, and A. L. Notkins (1972). In vitro stimulation of sensitized lymphocytes by herpes simplex virus and vaccinia virus. Proc. Nat. Acad. Sci. U.S.A. 69:756–760.
46. Rosenberg, G. L., C. Wohlenberg, A. J. Nahmias, and A. L. Notkins (1972). Differentiation of type 1 and type 2 herpes simplex virus by in vitro stimulation of immune lymphocytes. J. Immunol. 109:413–414.
47. Shapiro, A. L., E. Vinuela, and J. V. Maizel (1967). Molecular weight estimation of polypeptide chains by electrophoresis in SDS—polyacrylamide gels. Biochem. Biophys. Res. Commun. 23:815–820.
48. Spear, P. G. and B. Roizman (1972). Protein specified by herpes simplex virus. V. Purification and structural proteins of the herpesvirion. J. Virol. 9:143–159.
49. Stevens, J. G. and M. L. Cook (1974). Maintenance of latent herpetic infection: An apparent role of antiviral IgG. J. Immunol. 113:1685–1693.
50. Taverne, J. J., J. H. Marshall, and F. Fulton (1958). The purification and concentration of viruses and virus soluble antigens on calcium phosphate. J. Gen. Microbiol. 19:451–641.
51. Weber, K. and M. Osborn (1969). The reliability of molecular weight determinations by dodecyl sulfate polyacrylamide gel electrophoresis. J. Biol. Chem. 244:4406–4412.
52. Wilton, J. M. A., L. Ivanyi, and T. Lehner (1972). Cell-mediated immunity in herpesvirus hominis infections. Br. Med. J. 248:723–726.
53. Sydiskis, R. J. and B. Roizman (1967). The disaggregation of host polyribosomes in productive and abortive infection with herpes simplex virus. Virology 32:678–686.
54. Thurman, G. B., D. M. Strong, A. Ahmed, S. S. Green, K. W. Sell, R. J. Hertzman, and F. M. Bach (1973). Human mixed lymphocyte cultures. Evaluation of a microculture technique utilizing the multiple automated sample harvester (MASH). Clin. Exp. Immunol. 15:289–302.

CHAPTER 6

Epstein-Barr Virus: A Natural Latent Human Herpesvirus

B. Hampar[1] and J. G. Derge

I. INTRODUCTION

The EB virus is the only human herpesvirus shown to be capable of forming a natural latent infection in which the complete virus genome persists in a repressed form in replicating human cells (*21, 27*). Latency by EB virus appears to be limited to lymphoid cells of the B type, although persistence of the virus in nonlymphoid cells has been reported (*22*). In the case of carcinoma of the postnasal space, for example, the virus apparently persists in epitheloid-type cells, although the possibility that these cells may represent lymphoid precursor cells has not been excluded (*18, 26*).

The EB virus is similar to other herpesviruses in that it contains DNA of molecular weight of approximately 10^8 daltons. Lymphoblastoid cells latently infected with EB virus may contain up to 50 or more copies of the complete virus genome, which represents up to 0.1% of the total cell DNA (*21, 27*). The majority of these

[1]Viral Carcinogenesis Branch, National Cancer Institute, National Institutes of Health, Bethesda, Maryland 20014, and Flow Laboratories, Inc., Rockville, Maryland 20852.

Abbreviations: EB virus, Epstein-Barr virus; EBNA, EB virus nuclear antigen; EA, EB virus early antigen; VCA, EB virus structural antigen; BrdU, 5-bromodeoxyuridine; IdU, 5-iododeoxyuridine; P3HR-1(BU) cells, P3HR-1 cells made resistant to BrdU; dTK, thymidine kinase; dT, thymidine; HAT, selective medium containing hyposanthine, aminopterin, and dT; ara-C, 1-B-D-arabinofuranosylcytosine; HU, hydroxyurea; dCyt, deoxycytidine; Ade, adenine.

virus copies exist in a "plasmid" form and are not covalently bonded by DNA–DNA linkage to the cell DNA (1, 24). The possibility that one or more virus genome copies may actually be integrated into cell DNA has not been excluded and seems a likely possibility.

Activation of the EB virus genome may occur spontaneously in producer cells, while nonproducer cells show little or no evidence of spontaneous activation although they may contain more copies of the virus genome than producer cells. Similar to type C RNA viruses, activation of the repressed EB virus genome may be effected by incorporation of halogenated pyrimidines into DNA (4, 9).

The characteristics of the EB virus-human lymphoblastoid cell system that have relevance here may be briefly summarized as follows. Three intracellular antigen complexes detectable by immunofluorescence have been described in EB virus infected cells. The EB virus nuclear antigen (EBNA) is detected by immunofluorescent complement-fixation in nuclei of cells carrying a repressed or activated virus genome (23) and displays properties characteristic of the T antigens associated with DNA tumor viruses. The EBNA complex is found associated with cell chromatin material. The remaining two complexes are found in productively infected cells where the virus genome has been activated either spontaneously or after treatment with drugs. These include the early antigen (EA) complex, which represents virus products synthesized prior to productive replication of the virus DNA and which contains a restricted (R) and diffuse (D) component (17). The nature of the antigens comprising the EA complex (e.g., structural or nonstructural) is unknown. The second intracellular antigen complex contains virus structural antigens (VCA) and represents products synthesized subsequent to productive replication of the virus DNA (15).

Cells latently infected with EB virus may be classified into two types. Producer cells are those in which activation of the virus genome occurs spontaneously, giving rise to the synthesis of EA, VCA, and virus particles. Nonproducer cells are those in which spontaneous virus activation occurs rarely, and the activated cells synthesize EA but not VCA.

II. VIRUS PRODUCTIVE CYCLE IN SPONTANEOUSLY ACTIVATED CELLS

The events following spontaneous activation of the repressed EB virus genome have been studied in producer P3HR-1 cells and in P3HR-1 cells made resistant to BrdU: P3HR-1(BU) cells.

The P3HR-1(BU) cells are developed by exposing P3HR-1 cells to increasing concentrations of BrdU over a 6-month period (8). The drug-resistant cells show low but consistent levels of the enzyme dTK, suggesting that resistance to BrdU is not complete, although the cells grow well in the presence of BrdU concentrations of 100 μg/ml or more. This apparent discrepancy can be resolved by autoradiographic analysis, which indicates that the uptake of [^{3}H]dT is restricted to only a few cells in the population, in contrast to all cells showing low levels of incorporation as would be expected for a leaky mutant. Subsequent studies employing immunofluorescence in conjunction with autoradiography indicate that dTK activity in the P3HR-1(BU) cell population is limited to those cells in which the virus genome has activated spontaneously.

The properties of the P3HR-1(BU) cells were studied in detail with the following findings. First, the absence of dTK enzyme in nonactivated cells is absolute and no evidence of spontaneous reversion was observed over a 2-year period. Second, the cells cannot replicate efficiently in the presence of selective HAT medium. When maintained on the selective medium for prolonged periods, however, HAT-resistant cell lines still lack dTK enzyme but acquire resistance to aminopterin. Third, repeated efforts to identify the dTK that appears in P3HR-1(BU) cells as being other than cellular in nature were unsuccessful, suggesting that the enzyme may represent a depressed cellular enzyme rather than a viral coded enzyme. Similar conclusions have been obtained with somatic cell hybrids activated by IdU (14). Fourth, the properties of the P3HR-1(BU) cells were reproduced in three additional EB virus positive cell lines made resistant to BrdU. Two of these lines are the nonproducer NC-37 and Raji lines, both of which show evidence of VCA and virus particle production following development of resistance to BrdU. This differs dramatically from results with wild type NC-37 or Raji cells, where treatment for short periods with IdU or BrdU results in the synthesis of EA, but not VCA (5). Finally, when an EB virus negative T cell-like lymphoblastoid line is made resistant to BrdU, the resultant cells show no evidence of dTK and no survival potential in selective HAT medium, suggesting that the dTK which appears in the EB virus positive BrdU-resistant cell lines is related to the presence of the virus genome.

The sequence of EB virus synthesis in P3HR-1(BU) cells

following spontaneous activation was studied. Using a combination of immunofluorescence and autoradiographic techniques it was shown that EA is synthesized before the appearance of a functional dTK enzyme, while VCA synthesis follows the appearance of dTK enzyme (*10*). It was also found that while ara-C and HU could effectively inhibit cell DNA synthesis in nonactivated cells, DNA synthesis in EA positive cells is refractory to normally inhibitory concentrations of HU although still sensitive to inhibition by ara-C (*10, 20*).

The DNA synthesized in P3HR-1(BU) cells was studied using a double labeling technique employing [³H]dT and either [¹⁴C]dCyt or [¹⁴C]Ade (*2, 8*). Incorporation of dT was limited to virus activated cells while incorporation of dCyt or Ade into DNA occurred in all cells in the population. The results indicate that incorporation of [³H]dT in virus activated cells occurs in both cellular and viral DNA, suggesting that some cell DNA is synthesized in the EA positive P3HR-1(BU) cells in conjunction with productive replication of virus DNA. Similar studies were carried out in the presence of HU (*2, 10*) with essentially the same results in that both cell DNA and free virus DNA were synthesized. However, the cell DNA from both P3HR-1 and P3HR-1(BU) cells labeled in the presence of HU apparently represents sequences rich in G-C residues since it bands at a higher density than normal human DNA.

The results discussed thus far indicate that following activation of the virus genome in P3HR-1(BU) cells, EA is synthesized and is followed by a period of DNA synthesis where dTK enzyme is present. This in turn is followed by the synthesis of VCA. Since productive replication of herpesvirus invariably leads to cell death, one would anticipate that the dTK + P3HR-1(BU) cells could not survive. This was tested as follows. The DNA in both P3HR-1 and P3HR-1(BU) cells is labeled with [³H]dCyt in the presence of 100 μg/ml of BrdU over a several-day period and the isolated DNAs are banded in neutral CsCl (*13*). The P3HR-1 cells show three distinct labeled DNA peaks, one banding at the density of normal human DNA, one banding at a density corresponding to human DNA with BrdU substituted in both strands of DNA, and an intermediate peak banding at a density corresponding to human DNA in which only one strand had been substituted with BrdU (confirmed in alkaline gradients). In contrast, the P3HR-1(BU) cell DNA shows only two labeled DNA peaks, one banding at the density of normal human DNA, and the other banding at the density of human DNA substituted in only one strand with BrdU. Consequently, while P3HR-1 cells could undergo two or more cycles of DNA synthesis in the presence of BrdU, the P3HR-1(BU) cells could undergo only one cycle of DNA synthesis in the presence of the analog.

Synthesis of VCA and virus particles may be prevented if DNA synthesis is blocked following the appearance of EA in activated cells (6, 10). In the case of P3HR-1(BU) cells, synthesis of EA is not affected when cells are maintained on high concentrations (> 20 μg/ml) of BrdU, while synthesis of VCA and virus particles are inhibited (8). This is consistent with the sequence of events discussed above, where EA appears before dTK and a cycle of DNA synthesis (in dTK^+ cells) is required for synthesis of VCA. The effect of continued maintenance of the cells on BrdU is effectively to block or to slow down DNA synthesis by incorporation of the analog into DNA (11). Following the removal of BrdU, VCA is evident within 24 hr and virus particles appear in approximately 4 days (8).

III. VIRUS PRODUCTIVE CYCLE IN DRUG ACTIVATED CELLS

Following the initial observation that halogenated pyrimidines could activate EB virus in human lymphoblastoid cells (4, 9), a series of experiments was carried out to elucidate the mechanism of activation by drugs and the sequence of events that occurred in the activated cells. Since virus activation by halogenated pyrimidines requires incorporation of the drug into DNA, we assumed that activation occurs during the cell's S phase. This is consistent with other findings that indicate that spontaneous virus activation in stationary phase P3HR-1(BU) cells could be inhibited by blocking DNA synthesis following resuspension of the cells in fresh growth medium (9). Studies were carried out employing cells synchronized by the double thymidine blocking technique to study the events in cells activated by the IdU (Figure 1).

The initial studies dealt with the question of whether activation required incorporation of the IdU during a specific period in the cell cycle. Producer EB-3 cells and nonproducer Raji cells are synchronized and are treated for 60-min intervals throughout the cell cycle with IdU at a concentration of 20 μg/ml. The results (11) indicate that maximum virus activation occurs when the analog is added to cultures 60 min after initiation of the S phase (S-1 period). In the

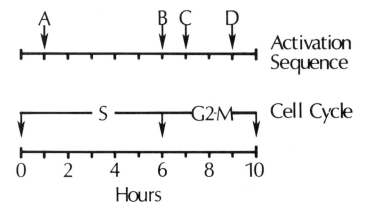

Figure 1. (*A*) Initiation of virus activation sequence; replication of repressed virus genome. (*B*) Synthesis of EA. (*B*)–(*C*) DNA synthesis required for VCA. (*D*) Synthesis of VCA.

case of producer EB-3 cells, approximately 50% of the activated cells progress to synthesis of VCA, while nonproducer Raji cells show synthesis of only EA.

The next series of experiments dealt with the question of whether replication of the resident EB virus genome occurred during a specific period in the cell cycle. Nonproducer Raji cells are synchronized and the cells are harvested at intervals for extraction of DNA and hybridization with virus specific complementary RNA (cRNA). The results (*14*) indicate that replication of the resident virus genome occurs between 30 and 90 min after initiation of the S phase, which corresponds to the critical time for IdU incorporation to induce virus activation. Based on these findings it was suggested that (1) virus activation is initiated near the site of association of the resident viral genome with cell DNA, (2) replication of the resident viral genome in nonactivated cells is under cell control mechanisms, and (3) the resident viral genome is physically associated with early replicating cell DNA.

Studies were carried out next to determine the sequence of antigen synthesis following activation by IdU. Synchronized cells are treated with IdU for 60 min starting 1 hr after reversal of the dT block and the cells are tested at intervals for antigen synthesis (*12*). The data may be summarized as follows. First, synthesis of EA occurs approximately 5 hr after removal of the IdU, which corresponds to the early G-2 period of the cell cycle. Synthesis of

VCA in producer EB-3 cells occurs approximately 3 hr after synthesis of EA. Second, inhibition of DNA synthesis by ara-C or HU added immediately after the 60-min treatment with IdU does not prevent the subsequent synthesis if EA, but does prevent the synthesis of VCA. The time of EA appearance in the ara-C or HU treated cells corresponds to the time of EA synthesis in cells devoid of drug and allows completion of the S phase. Consequently, while synthesis of EA occurs at a time that corresponds to the early G-2 period of the cell cycle, completion of the S phase is not required for synthesis of EA. Third, synthesis of VCA requires a critical period of DNA synthesis (approximately 1 hr), which occurs subsequent to completion of the cells' normal S phase and subsequent to the synthesis of EA. This period of DNA synthesis corresponds to the dTK positive DNA synthesis observed in spontaneously activated P3HR-1(BU) cells. Fourth, although IdU-activated nonproducer Raji cells cannot progress beyond EA synthesis in the virus productive cycle, the synthesis of EA, which is sufficient to ensure cell death (3), does not preclude the cells from undergoing very low levels of DNA synthesis and reaching mitosis where the chromosomes show positive staining for EA. The inability of the activated Raji cells to synthesize VCA apparently is related to their failure to undergo the critical period of DNA synthesis subsequent to the synthesis of EA. This critical period of DNA synthesis is required for productive replication of virus DNA and synthesis of VCA. It is of interest in this respect that somatic cell hybrids of Raji cells and human D-98 cells show synthesis of VCA and virus particles following short-term treatment with IdU, indicating that cellular control mechanisms rather than a defective virus genome are responsible for the aborted virus cycle in Raji cells (7). Fifth, the inability of all IdU-activated EB-3 cells to progress to VCA synthesis is attributed to the toxic effects of the incorporated IdU. Following the incorporation of IdU during the S-1 period, the cells are able to complete the S phase, but only approximately 50% of the cells are able to successfully divide and enter a second S phase. Consequently, the toxic effects of the IdU are manifested subsequent to completion of the S phase during which the analog is incorporated. The percentage of IdU treated cells unable to divide approximates the percentage of activated EB-3 cells unable to enter the critical period of DNA synthesis subsequent to EA synthesis and unable to synthesize VCA.

Drugs other than halogenated pyrimidines have been used to activate EB virus. In synchronized cells, inhibitors of protein synthesis (cycloheximide or puromycin) or removal of arginine (16) from the medium can result in activation. For activation to occur, however, the protein inhibitor must be added to the cultures during the S-1 period of the cell cycle at a time that corresponds to the critical period for IdU incorporation to initiate the virus activation sequence. In addition, activation by protein inhibitors requires that the inhibitor be removed after 5 hr. Consequently, the period of cycloheximide treatment for maximum activation to occur is localized from 1 to 6 hr after initiation of the S phase. The time of removal of the protein inhibitor corresponds to the time of EA synthesis in IdU-activated cells. Further, during the 1–6-hr treatment with cycloheximide, inhibition of DNA synthesis by ara-C or HU prevents the subsequent synthesis of EA or VCA, suggesting that DNA synthesis has to continue during the period of protein inhibition. This requirement for continued DNA synthesis is somewhat surprising, since the addition of cycloheximide alone results in approximately 85% inhibition of DNA synthesis during the 1–6-hr treatment period. Similar results were obtained when arginine deficiency was employed for activation.

The above findings raise the possibility that activation induced by inhibitors of protein synthesis or arginine deprivation may result partly from the inhibitory effect of the drug on cell DNA synthesis rather than from inhibition of protein synthesis alone. This was tested with HU at various concentrations with the following findings. When a concentration of HU is employed that inhibits DNA synthesis by approximately 85% during the period 1–6 hr after initiation of the S phase, virus activation occurs at levels comparable to those observed with arginine deficiency (4–6%) and approximately one-third of those observed with cycloheximide (12–15%). The time of HU treatment (1–6 hr after initiation of the S phase) for maximum activation to occur corresponds to the times observed with cycloheximide and arginine deficiency. It would appear that in the case of arginine deficiency at least, activation may be due to the inhibitory effect of the deficiency on DNA synthesis rather than to its effect on protein synthesis. In contrast, activation by cycloheximide probably involves inhibition of some required protein in addition to inhibition of DNA synthesis.

IV.   SEQUENCE OF EVENTS IN VIRUS ACTIVATED CELLS

Figure 2 summarizes the sequence of events we propose occurs in EB virus-activated cells. The sequence was derived from results

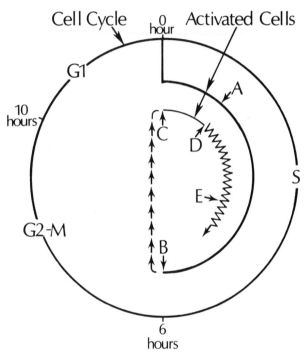

Figure 2. Proposed sequence of EB virus activation. Outer circle shows periods in the cell cycle of synchronized cultures. The short G-1 period is typical of synchronized cells and is probably artificially shortened in comparison to the length of this period in nonsynchronized cultures. Inner circles show events in virus activated cells. Virus activation is initiated during the S-1 period (A) at a time corresponding to the time of replication of the repressed virus genome. The cells progress through the S phase and EA is synthesized during the early G-2 period (B). The EA positive cells then initiate a new cycle of DNA synthesis (C) comparable to a "normal" S phase. In contrast to a normal S phase, however, this new cycle of DNA synthesis appears to be under control of the virus as evidenced by the following. First, the new cycle of DNA synthesis is refractory to normally inhibitory concentrations of HU, and second a dTK enzyme appears during this cycle that probably represents derepression of a cellular enzyme. The new cycle of DNA synthesis proceeds through the S phase for approximately 1 hr, when it again reaches the point of replication of the repressed virus DNA (D). Subsequent to reaching point (D), productive replication of virus DNA is initiated and this is followed shortly by synthesis of VCA (E).

obtained with spontaneously activated P3HR-1(BU) cells and drug-activated synchronized producer EB-3 cells and nonproducer Raji cells.

Virus activation is initiated during the S-1 period of the cell cycle at a time that approximates the time of replication of the resident virus genome (Figure 2, *A*). The mechanism of virus activation is somehow related to a disturbance in DNA synthesis, which probably alters the physical association between cell DNA and the resident viral DNA. This is suggested in the case of IdU treatment, where incorporation of the drug for a period as short as 30 min can result in activation, thus excluding the possibility that activation requires a mutagenic alteration in base pair sequences.

Synthesis of EA occurs approximately 5 hr after initiation of the activation sequence (Figure 2, *B*) at a time corresponding to the early G-2 period of the cell cycle. The 5-hr interval between the time of initiation of the activation sequence and synthesis of EA is predetermined and appears fixed regardless of the drug used for activation. The findings are consistent with the proposal that EA synthesis is related to synthesis of some cellular protein(s) during the early G-2 period, and that synthesis of EA and this G-2 protein(s) occurs at a fixed time regardless of whether completion of the cells normal S phase is prevented by drugs. We may speculate that the mRNAs for the G-2 protein(s) and EA are transcribed from cellular DNA that replicates during the first hour of the S phase, since in cells treated with IdU the S phase was allowed to proceed for 1 hr before the analog was added and subsequent DNA synthesis was blocked.

Following synthesis of EA (Figure 2, *B*) producer cells undergo a 1-hr period of DNA synthesis that is required for subsequent synthesis of VCA. The findings in P3HR-1(BU) cells that the activated EA positive, dTK positive cells synthesized both cell DNA and virus DNA are consistent with the proposed sequence in Figure 2, which suggests that upon completion of the S phase and synthesis of EA (Figure 2, *B*), the cells initiate a new cycle of DNA synthesis (Figure 2, *C*), which progresses through the S phase for approximately 1 hr (Figure 2, *D*) to reach the point where replication of the resident virus genome normally occurs. When this point is reached (Figure 2, *D*), replication of the resident virus DNA is dissociated from cell DNA and productive replication of virus DNA is initiated and is followed by synthesis of VCA (Figure 2, *E*).

The dTK positive DNA synthesis in activated P3HR-1(BU) cells would correspond to the period of DNA synthesis extending from *C* to *D* in Figure 2. At some point during this period of DNA synthesis the cells become insensitive to the inhibitory effects of HU. Consequently, while the DNA synthesis that occurs during the activated cells normal S phase (*A* to *B* in Figure 2) appears to remain under cellular control mechanisms, the DNA synthesis that occurs subsequent to the appearance of EA appears to be under control of the virus genome. Synthesis of dTK during the normal cell cycle should occur during the early S phase (*19*). The dTK that appears in activated P3HR-1(BU) cells would appear to be synthesized during the early G-2 period. However, if the sequence proposed in Figure 2 is correct, then synthesis of dTK enzyme in activated cells would actually occur near the time of initiation of a new S phase (Figure 2, *C*) and would correspond to the expected time of synthesis of this enzyme.

LITERATURE CITED

1. Adams, A., T. Lindahl, and G. Klein (1973). Linear association between cellular DNA and Epstein-Barr virus DNA in a human lymphoblastoid cell line. Proc. Nat. Acad. Sci. U.S.A. 70:2888–2892.

2. Derge, J. G., S. L. Birkhead, T. Hemmaplardh, and B. Hampar (1974). DNA synthesis in cells activated for the Epstein-Barr virus. Second Int. Symp. on Oncogenesis and Herpesviruses, Nuremberg, Germany, in press.

3. Diehl, V., H. Wolf, H. Schulte-Holthausen, and H. zur Hausen (1972). Re-exposure of human lymphoblastoid cell lines to Epstein-Barr virus. Int. J. Cancer. 10:641–651.

4. Gerber, P. (1972). Activation of Epstein-Barr virus by 5-bromodeoxyuridine in "virus-free" human cells. Proc. Nat. Acad. Sci. U.S.A. 69:83–85.

5. Gerber, P. and S. Lucas (1972). Epstein-Barr virus associated antigens activated in human cells by 5-bromodeoxyuridine. Proc. Soc. Exp. Biol. Med. 141:431–435.

6. Gergely. L., G. Klein, and I. Ernberg (1971). The action of DNA antagonists on Epstein-Barr virus (EBV)-associated early antigen (EA) in Burkitt lymphoma lines. Int. J. Cancer 7:293–302.

7. Glaser, R. and M. Nonoyama (1974). Host cell regulation if induction of Epstein-Barr virus. J. Virol. 14:174–176.

8. Hampar, B., J. G. Derge, L. M. Martos, and J. L. Walker (1971). Persistence of a repressed Epstein-Barr virus genome in Burkitt lymphoma cells made resistant to 5-bromodeoxyuridine. Proc. Nat. Acad. Sci. U.S.A. 68:3185–3189.

9. Hampar, B., J. G. Derge, L. M. Martos, and J. L. Walker (1972). Synthesis of Epstein-Barr virus after activation of the viral genome in a "virus-negative" human lymphoblastoid cell (Raji) made resistant to 5-bromodeoxyuridine. Proc. Nat. Acad. Sci. U.S.A. 69:78–82.

10. Hampar, B., J. G. Derge, L. M. Martos, M. A. Tagamets, and M. A. Burroughs (1972). Sequence of spontaneous Epstein-Barr virus activation and selective DNA synthesis in activated cells in the presence of hybroxyurea. Proc. Nat. Acad. Sci. U.S.A. 69:2589–2593.

11. Hampar, B., J. G. Derge, L. M. Martos, M. A. Tagamets, S. -Y. Chang, and M. Chakrabarty (1973). Identification of a critical period during the S phase for activation of the Epstein-Barr virus by 5-iododeoxyuridine. Nature (New Biol.) 244:214–217.

12. Hampar, B., J. G. Derge, M. Nonoyama, S. -Y. Chang, M. A. Tagamets, and S. D. Showalter (1974). Programming of events in Epstein-Barr virus-activated cells induced by 5-iododeoxyuridine. Virology 62:71–89.

13. Hampar, B., J. G. Derge, A. Tanaka, and M. Nonoyama (1974). Sequence of Epstein-Barr virus productive cycle in human lymphoblastoid cells. Cold Spring Harbor Symp. Quant. Biol. Tumor Viruses, 39:811–815.

14. Hampar, B., A. Tanaka, M. Nonoyama, and J. G. Derge (1974). Replication of the resident repressed Epstein-Barr virus genome during the early S phase (S-1 period) of nonproducer Raji cells. Proc. Nat. Acad. Sci. U.S.A. 71:631–633.

15. Henle, G. and W. Henle (1966). Immunofluorescence in cells derived from Burkitt's lymphoma. J. Bacteriol. 91:1248–1256.

16. Henle, W. and G. Henle (1968). Effect of arginine-deficient media on the herpes-type virus associated with cultured Burkitt tumor cells. J. Virol. 2:182–191.

17. Henle, W., G. Henle, B. A. Zajac, G. Pearson, R. Waubke, and M. Scriba (1970). Differential reactivity of human serums with early antigens induced by Epstein-Barr virus. Science 169:188–190.

18. Klein, G., B. C. Giovanella, T. Lindahl, P. J. Fialkow, S. Singh, and J. S. Stehlin (1974). Direct evidence for the presence of Epstein-Barr virus DNA and nuclear antigen in malignant epithelial cells from patients with poorly differentiated carcinoma of the nasopharynx Proc. Nat. Acad. Sci. U.S.A. 71:4737–4741.

19. Lin, S. -S. and W. Munyon (1974). Expression of the viral thymidine kinase gene in herpes simplex virus-transformed L cells. J. Virol. 14:1199–1208.

20. Mele, J., R. Glaser, M. Nonoyama, J. Zimmerman, and F. Rapp (1974). Observations on the resistance of Epstein-Barr virus DNA synthesis to hydroxyurea. Virol. 62:102–111.

21. Nonoyama, M. and J. S. Pagano (1971). Detection of Epstein-Barr viral genome in nonproductive cells. Nature (New Biol.) 233: 103–106.

22. Pattengale, P. K., R. W. Smith, and P. Gerber (1973). Selective transformation of B lymphocytes by EB virus. Lancet 2:93–94.

23. Reedman, B. and G. Klein (1973). Cellular localization of an Epstein-Barr virus (EBV)-associated complement-fixing antigen in producer and nonproducer lymphoblastoid cell lines. Int. J. Cancer 11:499–520.

24. Tanaka, A. and M. Nonoyama (1974). Latent DNA of Epstein-Barr virus: Separation from high molecular-weight cell DNA in a neutral glycerol gradient. Proc. Nat. Acad. Sci. U.S.A. 71:4658–4661.

25. Walboomers, J. M. M. and R. Glaser (1975). Thymidine kinase in Burkitt lymphoblastoid somatic cell hybrids after induction of the EB virus, in preparation.

26. Wolf, H., H. zur Hausen, and V. Becker (1973). EB viral genomes in epithelial nasopharyngeal carcinoma cells. Nature (New Biol.) 244:245–247.

27. zur Hausen, H. and H. Schulte-Holthausen (1970). Presence of EB virus nucleic acid homology in a "virus-free" line of Burkitt tumor cells. Nature (London) 227:245–248.

CHAPTER 7

Cell-Mediated Immunity In Murine Virus Tumor Systems

R. B. Herberman, H. Kirchner,
H. T. Holden, M. Glaser, S. Haskill, and G. D. Bonnard

I. INTRODUCTION

Type C virus-induced tumors function as antigens in mice and particularly in rats, and they can evoke vigorous cell-mediated immune responses to tumor-associated or virus-associated antigens. Extensive in vitro studies of cell-mediated immune responses to virus-induced lymphomas and sarcomas have been done in mice and rats. Cellular immunity has been studied by measuring proliferation of lymphocytes upon culture with tumor cells and by use of a ^{51}Chromium release assay (CRA) for examining cytotoxicity.

In addition to eliciting these responses by primary and secondary immunizations in vivo, it has also been possible to generate secondary cytotoxic responses in vitro by exposure of immune cells to tumor cells. The characteristics of these cell-mediated immune responses have been examined in detail with a particular emphasis on the dynamics of the responses and their relationship to growth or regression of the tumor. The ultimate objective of this area of research is to determine the role of the various cell-mediated immune responses that can be measured in vitro in the resistance of the host against progressive tumor growth.

II. CHARACTERISTICS OF CELL-MEDIATED
IMMUNE RESPONSES TO MURINE SARCOMA VIRUS (MSV)

The MSV tumor system in mice has been extensively studied because it is very antigenic. It has been possible to induce tumors that grow transiently and then regress (mice with such tumors are designated regressors), and also tumors that grow progressively and kill the host (progressors). Thus the immunologic responses associated with these divergent patterns of tumor growth can be compared. Intramuscular inoculation of most stocks of MSV into C57BL/6 mice results in transient local tumor growth; the tumor reaches maximal size at about 10 days and then rapidly and completely regresses (20). The mice are then strongly resistant to challenge with virus or with leukemias induced by Friend, Rauscher, or Moloney viruses. In contrast to the usual regression of MSV tumors, progressive tumor growth can be induced by regular stocks of MSV in very young or in immunosuppressed mice, or by some stocks of MSV even in adult recipients.

In parallel with the common tumor-associated transplantation antigens (TATAs) between MSV and virus-induced leukemias, demonstrated by in vivo protection, mice inoculated with MSV also

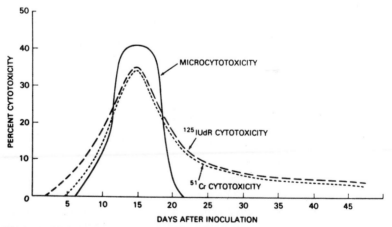

Figure 1. Measurement by three different assays of cell-mediated cytotoxic response of C57BL/6 mice at various times after inoculation with MSV. The CRA was performed 4 hr against RBL-5 target cells, at a 200:1 attacker to target (A/T) ratio. The IUdR assay and MCA were run for 48 hr against MSB target cells, with A/T ratios of 500–1,000:1 and 2,000–3,000:1, respectively.

develop cell-mediated immunity that can be detected in vitro with some leukemia target cells. Cell-mediated cytotoxicity, as measured by the reactivity of spleen cells against the Rauscher virus-induced leukemia RBL-5 in the 4-hr CRA (20), reaches a peak at about 14 days after MSV inoculation and then rapidly declines (Figure 1). Reactivity is distributed widely among the various lymphoid organs. The lymph nodes draining the site of virus inoculation become reactive very early, and this reactivity persists for a long period of time. Other lymph nodes, including the mesenteric nodes, peripheral blood lymphocytes, and peritoneal exudate cells develop cytotoxic reactivity with a time course similar to that in the spleen. Progressors have lower levels of reactivity, but the kinetics of response are very similar to those seen with regressors. The immune reactivity is T cell dependent, being abolished or markedly reduced by pretreatment with anti-θ plus complement (12). The antigen detected in this assay, designated MEV-SA1, is distinct from previously described serologic specificities, and is related to the expression of mouse endogenous type C viruses (11).

In addition to the CRA, specific cell-mediated cytotoxicity can also be measured by a visual microcytotoxicity assay (MCA) and by an [125]Iododeoxyuridine release assay (IUdR) (6). A summary of the results is shown in Figure 1. With the particular MSV target cell used for the MCA and IUdR assay, similar kinetics occur in all three assays, with peak responses at the same time. The only significant difference is the more rapid decline in cytotoxicity measured by the MCA. As with the CRA, reactivity in the other assays is eliminated by pretreatment of lymphocytes with anti-θ plus complement.

At 14 days after inoculation of MSV, spleen cells and peritoneal exudate cells inhibit the in vitro proliferation of RBL-5 tumor cells, as measured by incorporation of [^{3}H]thymidine (designated growth inhibition assay, GIA) (17, 19). In contrast to the other assays of cytotoxicity, the reactivity measured by GIA is nonspecific, with similar effects on a variety of tumor cells, including those negative for MEV-SA1. Also, the activity is not dependent on T cells. Macrophages appeared to be responsible for the activity, since the growth-inhibitory effects are removed or inactivated by treatment of effector cells with adherence columns, carbonyl iron and magnet, or with carrageenan (17, 19).

Primary MSV tumors have been described histologically as

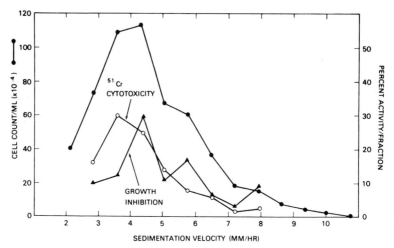

Figure 2. Separation of effector cells from primary MSV tumors, on Ficoll gradient by gravity sedimentation. The figure shows reactivity in CRA and GIA, calculated as the percent activity per fraction, and also the number of cells per milliliter recovered in each 40-ml fraction.

reactive granulomas, since they contain many normal mononuclear cells, including lymphocytes and macrophages (*28*). Cells active in both the CRA and GIA can be consistently recovered from MSV tumors (Figure 2). The cells reactive in CRA are small, with a sedimentation velocity of 3.5 mm/hr. The growth inhibitory cells appear to be somewhat larger and of a more heterogeneous population of cells, sedimenting more rapidly. The reactive cells within the primary tumors have somewhat different properties than the cells with those functions recovered from the spleen at the same time (Figure 3). In the spleen, the CRA reactive cells are larger and sediment at 5 mm/hr, and the growth inhibitory cells are slightly larger than the cytotoxic effector cells.

It appeared from early studies that only low levels of spleen cell cytotoxicity could be detected after regression of MSV tumors and that no rise in reactivity took place after secondary challenge with leukemia cells (*20, 21*). This cast some doubt on the in vivo relevance of the cytotoxicity assay, since the mice were strongly protected against growth of the leukemia cells. Recently, however, it has been shown that a secondary challenge elicits a rapid and vigorous cell-mediated cytotoxic response that is often confined to the region of challenge (*14*). After intramuscular challenge, the

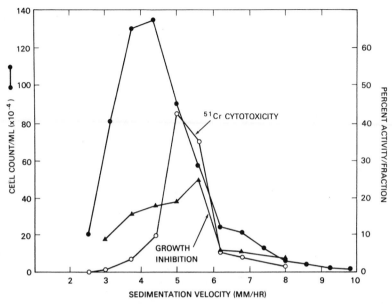

Figure 3. Separation of effector cells from spleens of C57BL/6 bearing primary MSV tumors, on Ficoll gradient by gravity sedimentation. The figure shows reactivity in CRA and GIA, calculated as the percent activity per fraction, and also the number of cells per milliliter recovered in each 40-ml fraction.

draining lymph node cells develop cytotoxic reactivity, and after intraperitoneal challenge, the peritoneal exudate cells become highly active. In many instances, particularly when challenge is more than 4 months after primary immunization, little or no cytotoxic reactivity can be detected in lymphoid organs that are distant from the site of challenge. The ability of immune mice to develop a rapid and strong cytotoxic response in the region of tumor growth may be a critical element in the resistance to tumor growth. The secondary cytotoxic response, like the primary response, appears to be mediated by T cells; treatment with anti-θ plus complement removes most of the cytotoxic reactivity.

It has also been possible in this system to begin to analyze in vitro the steps in antigen recognition and generation of cytotoxic lymphocytes. In mixed cultures of lymphocytes with RBL-5 cells, normal mice usually show no detectable proliferative response. Low levels of significant proliferation have been detected in regressors, but only during a brief period, at about 14 days after MSV inoculation.

In contrast, incubation of RBL-5 cells with lymphocytes from immune mice, obtained over a wide period of time after MSV inoculation, produces high levels of cytotoxic reactivity. This in vitro generated secondary cytotoxic response is specific and appears to be mediated by T cells.

III. CHARACTERISTICS OF CELL-MEDIATED IMMUNE RESPONSE TO GROSS VIRUS-INDUCED TUMOR IN RATS

The Gross virus-induced lymphoma (C58NT)D in W/Fu rats is highly antigenic and usually produces transiently growing tumors that then regress. However, progressors can be produced by inoculation of very high numbers of cells (greater than 1×10^8) or by immunosuppression. After regression of (C58NT)D, rats remain resistant to rechallenge with even high doses of tumor cells, for periods of over 1 year. Cytotoxic lymphocytes, as measured by CRA, are found early after tumor cell inoculation; the activity in the spleen reaches a peak in about 10 days and then declines to low levels or becomes undetectable by 20 days (23). The same pattern of activity is found in regressors or progressors; the progressors, however, have lower peak activity. The primary cytotoxic reactivity in the CRA is dependent on T cells, and can be eliminated by treatment with specific anti-T cell serum plus complement (5). As in the MSV system, reactivity after tumor cell inoculation appears earlier in draining lymph nodes than in the spleen (24). Peripheral blood lymphocytes and peritoneal exudate cells also show reactivity, with kinetics very similar to those seen with spleen cells. Direct cytotoxicity is not found in any of the lymphoid organs after regression of tumor. However, lymphocytes from rats 35 days or more after tumor inoculation are activated after incubation at 37°C for 12–24 hr (25). The cytotoxicity produced by the activated cells appears to be mediated by non-T cells, since it is not affected by treatment with specific anti-T cell serum plus complement. When cytotoxic reactivity is measured in the MCA, results are found early after tumor inoculation and at 40–120 days (29). This assay involves a 40–48 hr incubation period, sufficient time for activation of lymphocytes. As in the MSV tumor system, analysis of the specificity of the cell-mediated cytotoxic reactions shows that the detected antigens are quite distinct from any of those detected by humoral antibodies (26). The antigens appear to be related to expression of rat endogenous type C virus (22).

As in the MSV tumor system, it has been possible to induce a secondary cytotoxic response by rechallenge of immune rats with (C58NT)D tumor cells. A rapid and strong response is detectable, both in the region of challenge and to a lesser extent, in other lymphoid organs. In contrast to the transitory nature of the secondary cytotoxic response in the MSV tumor system, cells in the region of challenge remain reactive for long periods of time.

Cell-mediated immunity in this system can be measured by the proliferative response of lymphocytes to tumor cells (8). Lymphocytes from normal rats give no detectable responses. Significant proliferation of lymphocytes from regressors is detected at times when cytotoxic reactivity already is declining or has disappeared; it first is seen at 14 days after tumor inoculation, reaches a peak at days 20–40, and gradually declines to low levels by day 90 (Figure 4). With progressively growing tumors, there is no lymphocyte proliferation. As in the MSV tumor system, the in vitro incubation of lymphocytes from regressors with tumor cells also leads to a secondary generation of highly cytotoxic lymphocytes. The cytotoxic response is very rapid, occurring by 2 days of culture, in contrast to the proliferation assay in which activity first is detectable at 3 days. Another point of contrast with the proliferation assay is the ability to generate strong cytotoxic reactivity with cells obtained from rats 6–9 months after primary inoculation of (C58NT)D (by which time no proliferative response was detectable).

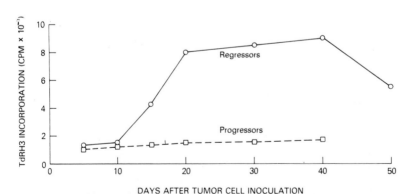

Figure 4. Proliferative response to mitomycin C treated (C58NT)D cells of spleen cells from regressors (○) or from progressors (□) tested at various times after inoculation of 1×10^9 (C58NT)D tumor cells. The results are expressed as mean counts per minute (cpm) of tritiated thymidine (TdRH3) of triplicate cultures.

IV. LYMPHOID CELLS CAUSING
SUPPRESSION OF CELL-MEDIATED IMMUNITY

One of the current critical questions in tumor immunology is: Why do tumors frequently grow progressively despite the ability of the host to mount an immune response against the tumors? Most of the recent studies have been concerned with the possible role of humoral factors in interfering with, or abrogating, effective cell-mediated immunity. Of particular interest have been "serum blocking factors" (2). In the two tumor systems described above, it is pertinent to consider the factors that contribute to progressive tumor growth. We have noted some defects in the cell-mediated immune responses in the progressors, i.e., decreased levels of cytotoxic activity, and undetectable proliferative response to the (C58NT)D. In trying to analyze the mechanisms for these defects, it is apparent that factors other than humoral were involved. One such factor is the inhibition of cellular immunity by suppressor cells. It was initially noted that mice bearing MSV-induced tumors have a markedly depressed lymphocyte proliferative response to phytohemagglutinin (PHA) (15, 16). In regressors, this depression is observed only transiently, at the time of peak tumor size. In progressors, the PHA response is defective throughout the entire growth period of the tumor. The depressed PHA response could be attributed to the suppressive effects of a subpopulation of spleen cells, rather than to an intrinsic deficit in PHA responsive T cells. Addition of spleen cells from MSV tumor-bearing mice to cultures of normal spleen cells results in a marked inhibition of PHA response (15). The suppressor cells have the characteristics of macrophages. They are removed or inactivated by treatment with carbonyl iron and magnet or with carrageenan or by passage through rayon adherence columns, and are unaffected by treatment with anti-θ plus complement, 4,000 R x-irradiation, or by passage through an anti-immunoglobulin immunoabsorbent column. Lymphocyte responses to concanavalin A are also markedly depressed in tumor-bearing mice (16). Reactivity to bacterial lipopolysaccharide, a B-cell mitogen, is affected to a lesser degree, and reactivity to pokeweed mitogen is not significantly depressed. Responses of spleen cells from MSV tumor-bearing mice in mixed leukocyte cultures with allogeneic cells are also deficient. All of the depressed responses have been shown to be due to the action of suppressor cells. Of particular relevance

here is the observation that the weak response in MLTI of spleen
cells from regressors at 14 days after MSV inoculation can be
considerably augmented by passage of the cells over a rayon adherence column, a procedure known to remove suppressor cells (19).
In some instances, a borderline or negative proliferative reaction
can be made clearly positive by such treatment (19).

The role of suppressor cells in depressing lymphocyte proliferation in response to tumor cells has been seen more strikingly in the
(C58NT)D tumor system. As noted above, progressors never have
detectable proliferative reactions to tumor cells. They also have poor
responsiveness to PHA. However, passage of spleen cells from progressors over rayon adherence columns restores PHA responsiveness,
and the nonadherent cells are quite reactive to tumor cells (9). The
role of suppressor cells can be documented by the addition of cells
from progressor rats to the mixture of tumor cells with regressor
cells (Figure 5). This results in a strong inhibition of the proliferative response of the immune, regressor cells, clearly indicating
that lymphocytes from rats bearing progressively growing tumors
do have the ability to recognize and be stimulated in vitro by tumor
cells, but that their proliferative response is abrogated by suppressor
cells.

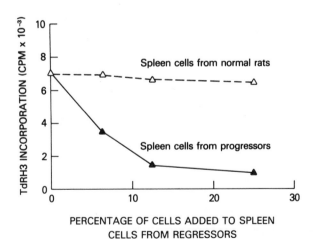

Figure 5. Inhibition of proliferative response of regressor lymphocytes to
(C58NT)D, by spleen cells from progressors. To a mixture of spleen cells
from regressors and mitomycin C treated (C58NT)D cells, varying propor-
tions of spleen cells from progressors (▲) or from normal rats (△)
were added.

All of the effects of the suppressor cells described thus far involve inhibition of proliferation of lymphocytes, particularly T cells. The suppressor cells and the effector cells in the GIA, involving inhibition of proliferation of tumor cells, have the same characteristics, and it seems quite likely that the same cells are responsible for both activities. If this is the case, there is the paradoxical potential that the same cells have opposing effects on tumor growth. On the one hand, the cells can inhibit growth of tumor cells, and on the other hand, they can interfere with cellular immunity against the tumor. However, this interference with cellular immunity has not been complete. The suppressor cells have no effect on the cytotoxicity in CRA by mice previously immunized to MSV (*15, 19*). In contrast to this inability to affect cytotoxicity by previously sensitized effector cells, the suppressor cells can interfere with the secondary generation in vitro of cytotoxic cells. Spleen cells prepared from mice at 14 days after MSV inoculation and pretreated with anti-θ plus complement to remove cytotoxic T cells, were added to cultures of RBL-5 and spleen cells from regressors obtained 30 days after inoculation with MSV. As shown in Table 1, the spleen cells from the MSV tumor-bearing mice inhibited the appearance of cytotoxic cells.

Suppressor cells also inhibit the in vivo secondary cytotoxic response of mice to tumor cells. In these experiments, it is logistically easier to use spleen cells from mice treated 14 days earlier with *Corynebacterium parvum* as the source of suppressor cells, since these cells lack detectable cytotoxic activity against RBL-5 in CRA. Suppressor cells induced by *C. parvum* have essentially the same characteristics as those induced by tumor growth (*18*). Challenge of MSV immune mice with a mixture of x-irradiated RBL-5 cells and spleen cells from *C. parvum* treated mice results in a much lower secondary cytotoxic response than that seen when mice are challenged with RBL-5 cells mixed with normal spleen cells (Table 2).

V. SERUM-MEDIATED
INHIBITION OF CELL-MEDIATED IMMUNITY

The MSV tumor system was the first in which specific blocking of colony inhibition and microcytotoxicity assays by serum was shown (*10*). Serum also has been reported to specifically block cytotoxicity

Table 1. Inhibition in vitro of secondary cytotoxic response to RBL-5 tumor cells by spleen cells from mice bearing MSV-inducted tumors

Source of added supressor cells[a]	% Cytotoxicity[b]	
	Immune spleen cells alone[c]	Immune spleen cells + RBL-5[d]
None	9.1	33.5
MSV tumor-bearer[e]	1.8	14.0
Normal mouse	1.5	29.6

[a]20×10^6 spleen cells, after pretreatment with anti-θ plus complement, were added to immune cells prior to culture.

[b]At end of culture, effector cells tested against RBL-5 ascites tumor cells, at ratio of 50:1.

[c]Immune spleen cells were obtained from C57BL/6 regressors, 30 days after MSV inoculation. 20×10^6 cells were placed in culture for 5 days.

[d]RBL-5 ascites tumor cells, pretreated with 100 μg/ml of mitomycin C for 30 min, at 1:30 ratio to immune spleen cells, were added before culture for 5 days.

[e]C57BL/6 mice, 14 days after inoculation of MSV.

Table 2. Inhibition in vivo of secondary cytotoxic response to x-irradiated RBL-5 tumor cells by spleen cells from mice pretreated with C. parvum

	Treatment of mice immunized 40 days before with MSV	
None	RBL-5 cells + normal spleen cells[a]	RBL-5 cells + spleen cells from C. parvum treated mice[b]
3.8(0.2)[c]	16.0(0.8)[c]	5.4(0.1)[c]
	17.3(0.3)	6.8(0.4)
	34.0(0.6)	7.9(0.5)
	16.4(0.2)	8.9(0.3)
	30.4(0.5)	

[a]1×10^6 RBL-5, irradiated with 5,000 R, were mixed with 1×10^8 spleen cells from normal C57BL/6 mice, and inoculated intraperitoneally.

[b]1×10^6 RBL-5, irradiated with 5,000 R, were mixed with 1×10^8 spleen cells from C57BL/6, inoculated 14 days earlier with 2.1 mg of heat-killed C. parvum and inoculated intraperitoneally.

[c]Percent cytotoxicity ($\pm$ standard error) against RBL-5 ascites target cells, of spleen cells from mice 4 days after intraperitoneal challenge of experimental groups with RBL-5 cells. The cells from the unchallenged controls were tested as a pool, whereas the spleen cells of challenged mice were tested individually.

in the CRA against (C58NT)D (27). However, in CRA, normal mouse or rat sera frequently inhibit cell-mediated cytotoxicity, and significant specific inhibition above this level by serum from tumor-bearing individuals has not been consistently observed. In studies of the mechanism of in vitro activation of cytotoxicity of W/Fu rat cells 40 days or more after inoculation of (C58NT)D, sera from rats previously inoculated with tumor cells inhibit this activation significantly more than do normal sera (25). However, these results are not clear-cut, since at the high levels of immune sera needed to achieve complete inhibition, normal rat sera also have some inhibitory effects.

Serum factors from tumor-bearing rats also inhibit lymphocyte stimulation. Addition of sera from rats with progressor (C58NT)D tumors inhibits the lymphoproliferative response to tumor cells of regressors (9). This inhibition by serum is not specific, since lymphocyte stimulation by PHA is also inhibited. One possible type of nonspecific inhibitory factor that is elevated in the sera of tumor-bearing individuals is immunoregulatory α-globulin (4). A preparation of α-globulin isolated from normal human plasma inhibits the MLTI of rats immune to (C58NT)D (7). However, since no elevated levels of α-globulins are found in the sera of tumor-bearing rats compared to normal rats, the role of this factor in the inhibition produced by progressor serum remains to be determined.

VI. INHIBITION OF CELL-MEDIATED IMMUNITY
BY TUMOR CELLS AND BY MATERIALS FROM TUMORS

Immunosuppression may also occur by action of the tumor itself or by products of the tumor. Only low concentrations of (C58NT)D cells cause proliferation of normal allogeneic or syngeneic immune lymphocytes, and this can be attributed to inhibitory properties of higher doses of the tumor cells (3). Addition of (C58NT)D cells to normal thymocytes results in a marked inhibition of the mixed leukocyte culture response to allogeneic normal cells. Similarly, certain doses of RBL-5 and other mouse ascitic lymphoma cells inhibit proliferation of normal lymphocytes (13). In order to demonstrate a positive MLTI in these systems or to generate in vitro secondary cytotoxic responses, it is necessary to determine carefully doses of tumor cells that are not inhibitory and that still possess sufficient stimulatory activity. One ascitic mouse lymphoma, EL-4, has two sublines, of which one is very strongly inhibitory and the other has only weak inhibitory properties. This allows a detailed analysis of the mechanisms of inhibition. EL-4 is a benzpyrene-induced lymphoma of C57BL mice that has been carried as a transplantable ascitic tumor for many years. Most of the current lines of EL-4 contain large amounts of endogenous type C virus and the Gross cell surface antigen (1, 11). Such sublines have been designated EL-4(G+). These cells also contain MEV-SA1 (11). In addition, there is a cryopreserved earlier passage of EL-4 that lacks Gross cell surface antigen and MEV-SA1, and has only low amounts of type C virus. This has been designated EL-4(G−). Both sublines at times contain some common murine viruses, e.g., lactic dehydrogenase virus, polyoma virus, and minute virus. A wide range of doses of EL-4(G+) cells can stimulate allogeneic Balb/c lymphocytes, although at the highest doses used no lymphocyte proliferation or generation of cytotoxic cells occurs (Figure 6). In contrast, generation of cytotoxic cells is only seen with very low doses of EL-4(G−) cells. The absence of reactivity is due to active inhibition by the EL-4(G−) ascites cells, as revealed by the low cytotoxic response in allogeneic mixed reactions in which

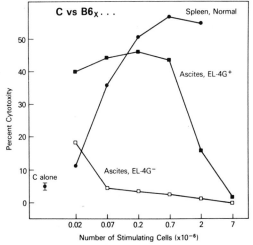

Figure 6. Failure to generate allogeneic cytotoxic reactivity by most doses of EL-4(G −) ascites cells and by the highest doses of EL-4(G +) ascites cells. 5 × 10⁶ BALB/c (C) spleen cells were incubated with varying doses of x-irradiated C57BL/6 (B6ₓ) normal spleen cells, EL-4(G −), or EL-4(G +). After 5 days, cytotoxicity against RBL-5 target cells was measured.

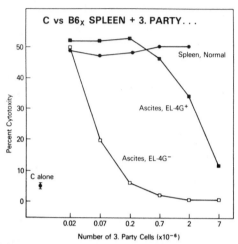

Figure 7. Inhibition of generation of allogeneic cytotoxicity by most doses of EL-4(G $-$) ascites cells and by the highest doses of EL-4(G $+$) ascites cells. To mixtures of 5×10^6 BALB/c (C) spleen cells and 2×10^6 irradiated C57BL/6 (B6$_x$) spleen cells were added varying numbers of the following third-party cells: normal C57BL/6 spleen cells, EL-4(G $+$), or EL-4(G $-$) ascites cells. After 5 days in culture, cytotoxicity against RBL-5 target cells was measured.

the EL-4(G$-$) cells are added as third-party cells (Figure 7). Inhibition also occurs when EL-4(G$-$) cells are added to the mixture of C57BL/6 cells and Balb/c stimulating cells.

Culture fluids of EL-4(G$-$) cells grown in vitro, particularly during the first 20 passages, after passage through a 0.22-μ filter, are strongly inhibitory. Results of studies performed to date have been consistent with the conclusion that the inhibition is due to a virus. Some of the relevant data are summarized in Figure 8. The supernatant of culture fluids of EL-4(G $-$) has no inhibitory activity, whereas the pellet, resuspended in a third of the original volume, is correspondingly more active. Culture fluid exposed to ultraviolet irradiation, loses its inhibitory activity. Finally, the inhibition by a given dilution of culture fluid is progressively abolished by increasing doses of cell-free ascites fluid from mice bearing the EL-4(G$-$) tumor. It seems likely that the ascites fluid contains antibodies that are able to inactivate the inhibitory agent. These data suggest the presence within some tumor cells of a virus that can inhibit proliferative and cytotoxic responses. However, further

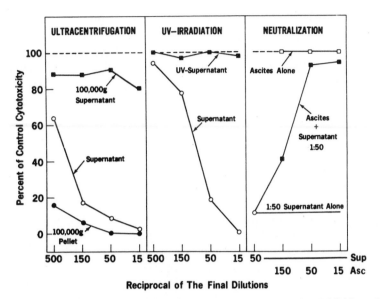

Figure 8. Evidence for the possible role of a virus in the inhibition, by products of tumor cells, of generation of allogeneic cytotoxic effector cells. To mixtures of BALB/c spleen cells and B6ₓ (as in Figure 7) were added varying dilutions of a culture fluid (supernatant) from EL-4(G —) cells. After 5 days in culture, cytotoxicity against RBL-5 target cells was measured. Control cytotoxicity, obtained in the mix without added supernatant, was normalized to 100%. *Left,* supernatant was centrifuged at 100,000 × g for 60 min and resultant pellet and supernatant added. *Center,* the culture fluid was tested after ultraviolet irradiation (UV-supernatant). *Right,* a 1:50 dilution of culture fluid was added alone (1:50 supernatant alone) or with various dilutions of a cell-free ascites fluid from mice bearing EL-4(G —) tumors. Various dilutions of ascites fluid alone were also tested as controls.

studies will be needed to determine the nature of this agent and its possible immunosuppressive role in vivo.

VII. CONCLUSIONS

The cell-mediated immune responses in the virus-induced tumor systems are quite complex, and one must be very cautious in directly relating in vitro data to in vivo effector mechanisms. Our data indicate that when various in vitro assays are used to measure the kinetics of the immune response to tumor-associated antigens, considerable differences are seen. In analyzing these reactions, it is necessary to consider the reactivity of different subpopulations of lymphoid cells, and the various phases of the immune response, against a variety of cell surface antigens. In addition, the immune status is neither stable nor homogeneous within the various lymphoid organs, but is affected by a variety of factors, particularly the pattern of tumor growth. The level of immunity detected in the spleen may not be as relevant to the in vivo immune status as the immune reactivity in the region of tumor growth or within the tumor itself. Reexposure of the animal to tumor antigens may evoke a rapid and vigorous secondary immune response of lymphoid cells in the region and may also cause a migration of memory cells to the site of challenge.

Of central importance in tumor immunology is the mechanism by which tumors can grow progressively despite the potential for a vigorous and effective immune response against the tumor. As shown in the tumor systems under study here, some phases of the immune response, i.e., proliferation of lymphocytes and generation of cyto-toxic effector cells, seem to be particularly sensitive to inhibition, and a variety of factors can cause depression of the cell-mediated immune responses. The depressive factors include suppressor cells, specific or nonspecific serum inhibitors, and products of the tumor cells them-selves. It will be of considerable interest to determine the possible relationships among the various forms of immunodepression. For example, it is conceivable that all of the apparently diverse inhibitory effects are due to a common mechanism. Viruses or other inhibitory factors might be released in vivo from tumor cells, circulate in the serum, and cause activation of suppressor cells. A series of experi-ments can now be designed to test this and other possibilities. It will be important, in a particular tumor system, to determine which, if any, of these inhibitory factors play the predominant role in pro-moting tumor growth.

LITERATURE CITED

1. Aoki, T., R. B. Herberman, J. W. Hartley, M. Liu, M. J. Walling, and M. Nunn (1975). Surface antigens on transplantable tumor cell lines producing mouse endogenous type C viruses. Submitted for publication.
2. Baldwin, R. W., M. J. Embleton, M. R. Price, and A. Robins (1974). Immunity in the tumor-bearing host and its modification by serum factors. Cancer 34:1452–1460.

3. Bonnard, G. D. and R. B. Herberman (1975). Suppression of lymphocyte proliferative responses by murine lymphoma cells. *In* A. S. Rosenthal (ed.), Immune Recognition, Academic Press, Inc., New York, p. 817–828.

4. Cooperband, S. R., A. M. Badger, R. C. Davis, K. Schmid, and J. A. Mannick (1972). The effect of immunoregulatory α-globulin (IRA) upon lymphocytes in vitro. J. Immunol. 109:154–163.

5. Djeu, J. Y., M. Glaser, H. Kirchner, K. Y. Huang, and R. B. Herberman (1974). The effect of specific anti-rat thymocyte serum on cell-mediated tumor immunity and other lymphocyte functions. Cell. Immunol. 12:164–169.

6. Fossati, G., H. T. Holden, and R. B. Herberman (1975). Evaluation of the cell-mediated immune response to murine sarcoma virus by [125]Iododeoxyuridine assay and comparison with [51]Chromium and microcytotoxicity assays. Cancer Res. 35:2600–2608.

7. Glaser, M. and R. B. Herberman (1974). The effect of immunoregulatory α-globulin (IRA) on in vitro proliferation of rat lymphocytes to syngeneic Gross virus-induced lymphoma. J. Nat. Cancer Inst. 53:1767–1769.

8. Glaser, M., R. B. Herberman, H. Kirchner, and J. Y. Djeu (1974). Study of the cellular immune response to Gross virus-induced lymphoma by the mixed lymphocyte-tumor interaction. Cancer Res. 34:2165–2171.

9. Glaser, M., H. Kirchner, and R. B. Herberman (1975). Inhibition of in vitro lymphoproliferative response to tumor associated antigens by progressively growing Gross virus-induced tumors. Int. J. Cancer 16:384–393.

10. Hellström, I. and K. E. Hellström (1969). Studies on cellular immunity and its serum mediated inhibition in Moloney-virus-induced mouse sarcomas. Int. J. Cancer 4:587–598.

11. Herberman, R. B., T. Aoki, M. Nunn, D. H. Lavrin, N. Soares, A. Gazdar, H. Holden, and K. S. S. Chang (1974). Specificity of ^{51}Cr-release cytotoxicity by lymphocytes immune to murine sarcoma virus. J. Nat. Cancer Inst. 53:1103–1111.

12. Herberman, R. B., M. E. Nunn, D. H. Lavrin, and R. Asofsky (1973). Effect of antibody to θ antigen on cell-mediated immunity induced in syngeneic mice by murine sarcoma virus. J. Nat. Cancer Inst. 51:1509–1512.

13. Herberman, R. R., C. C. Ting, H. Kirchner, H. Holden, M. Glaser, G. D. Bonnard, and D. Lavrin (1974). Effector mechanisms in tumour immunity. Prog. Immunol. II 3:285–295.

14. Holden, H. T., H. Kirchner, and R. B. Herberman (1975). Secondary cell-mediated cytotoxic response to syngeneic mouse tumor challenge. J. Immunol. 115:327–331.

15. Kirchner, H. T. M. Chused, R. B. Herberman, H. T. Holden, and D. H. Lavrin (1974). Evidence of suppressor cell activity in spleens of mice bearing primary tumors induced by Moloney sarcoma virus. J. Exp. Med. 139:1473–1487.

16.   Kirchner, H., R. B. Herberman, M. Glaser, and D. H. Lavrin (1974). Suppression of in vitro lymphocyte stimulation in mice bearing primary Moloney sarcoma virus-induced tumors. Cell. Immunol. 13:32–40.

17.   Kirchner, H., H. T. Holden, and R. B. Herberman (1975). Inhibition of in vitro growth of lymphoma cells by macrophages from tumor bearing mice. J. Nat. Cancer Inst. 55:971–975.

18.   Kirchner, H., H. T. Holden, and R. B. Herberman (1975). Splenic suppressor macrophages induced in mice by injection of *Corynebacterium parvum*. J. Immunol. 15:1212–1216.

19.   Kirchner, H., A. V. Muchmore, T. M. Chused, H. T. Holden, and R. B. Herberman (1975). Inhibition of proliferation of lymphoma cells and T lymphocytes by suppressor cells from spleens of tumor-bearing mice. J. Immunol. 114:206–210.

20.   Lavrin, D. H., R. B. Herberman, M. Nunn, and N. Soares (1973). In vitro cytotoxicity studies of murine sarcoma virus (MSV)-induced immunity in mice. J. Nat. Cancer Inst. 51:1497–1508.

21.   Leclerc, J. C., E. Gomard, and J. P. Levy (1972). Cell-mediated reaction against tumors induced by oncornaviruses. I. Kinetics and specificity of the immune response in murine sarcoma virus (MSV)-induced tumors and transplanted lymphomas. Int. J. Cancer 10:589–601.

22.   Nunn, M., J. Djeu, D. Lavrin, and R. B. Herberman (1976). Natural cytotoxic reactivity of rat lymphocytes against syngeneic Gross lymphoma. J. Nat. Cancer Inst., in press.

23.   Oren, M. E., R. B. Herberman, and T. G. Canty (1971). Immune response to Gross virus-induced lymphoma. II. Kinetics of the cellular immune response. J. Nat. Cancer Inst. 46:621–628.

24.   Ortiz de Landazuri, M. and R. B. Herberman (1972). Immune response to Gross virus-induced lymphoma. III. Characteristics of the cellular immune response. J. Nat. Cancer Inst. 49:147–154.

25.   Ortiz de Landazuri, M. and R. B. Herberman (1972). In vitro activation of cellular immune response to Gross virus-induced lymphoma. J. Exp. Med. 136:969–983.

26.   Ortiz de Landazuri, M. and R. B. Herberman (1972). Specificity of cellular immune reactivity to virus-induced tumors. Nature New Biol. 238:18–19.

27.   Shellam, G. R. and R. A. Knight (1974). Antigenic inhibition of cell-mediated cytotoxicity against tumour cells. Nature 252:330–332.

28.   Stanton, M., R. C. Ting, and L. W. Law (1968). Some biologic, immunogenic, and morphologic effects in mice after infection with a murine sarcoma virus. II. Morphologic studies. J. Nat. Cancer Inst. 40:1113–1129.

29.   Wright, P. W., M. Ortiz de Landazuri, and R. B. Herberman (1973). Immune response to Gross virus-induced lymphoma: Comparison of two in vitro assays of cell-mediated immunity. J. Nat. Cancer Inst. 50:947–954.

CHAPTER 8

Effects of Leukemia Viruses on Cell-Mediated Immune Responses

W. S. Ceglowski,
G. U. LaBadie, and A. A. Mascio

I. INTRODUCTION

Studies by numerous investigators in recent years have demonstrated that viruses, both oncogenic and nononcogenic, can affect the expression of host immune competence (*11, 13, 22, 25*). Such studies have provided information regarding humoral and cell-mediated immune mechanisms, viral immunopathogenesis, and the role of immune processes in the induction and maintenance of the neoplastic state. The increased knowledge of cell-mediated immune mechanisms and the enhanced awareness of its importance in tumor immunity stimulated the studies described in this chapter.

An early study by Dent, Petersen, and Good demonstrated that mice infected with Gross passage A virus exhibited a reduced capacity to reject skin grafts across a non-H-2-histocompatibility barrier (*10*). In contrast, Schneider and Dore reported that rejection of skin allografts in Friend leukemia virus-infected mice was comparable to that of noninfected controls (*26*). However, following reexamination of their data, Dent concluded that some impairment

Supported in part by Public Health Research Grant CA-15643 from the National Cancer Institute.

of graft rejection was actually observed (*11*). In related studies, Chirigos et al. have observed that infection of mice with Moloney leukemia virus, Rauscher leukemia virus, or Friend leukemia virus would effectively prevent the regression of Moloney sarcoma virus-induced tumors that is routinely observed in nonleukemia virus-infected control animals (*9*).

A study by Borella indicated that spleen cells from Rauscher leukemia virus-infected mice were capable of stimulation by phytohemagglutinin as measured by the incorporation of tritiated thymidine (*6*). However, the ratio of counts per minute in the presence of PHA to counts per minute in the absence of PHA was always lower than controls for the spleen cultures from infected animals. This was due in large part to the increased background incorporation in splenocytes from the Rauscher leukemia virus-infected mice. In contrast, Hayry, Rago, and Defendi, using an in vitro system, demonstrated a marked depression in the response of mouse splenocytes to PHA in the presence of Rauscher leukemia virus (*16*). Studies of preleukemic AKR mice as well as preleukemic C3H mice infected with Gross virus demonstrated significant impairment in the production of migration inhibitory factor in both groups of preleukemic mice when compared with appropriate controls (*12*). Others demonstrated that the several immunocompetent cell functions were unimpaired by infection with Friend leukemia virus (*3*). The thymic component in the response to sheep erythrocytes, antigen reactive cells, was not impaired. Also, both graft-versus-host reactivity and the proliferative capacity of "alloantigen-sensitive units" were not impaired by virus infection.

II.   EFFECT OF LEUKEMIA VIRUSES (FLV and RLV)

Our studies were done with either Friend leukemia virus (FLV) or Rauscher leukemia virus (RLV) as the oncogenic virus; these were selected primarily because they can rapidly induce a rather uniform disease state in susceptible adult mice. The BALB/c mouse was used in most experiments although the susceptible DBA/2 as well as the virus-resistant C57B1/6 mouse have also been used. As the parameters of cell-mediated immunity, we have utilized allograft rejection, macrophage migration inhibition (MMI), Concanavalin A stimulation, and lymphocyte-mediated cytotoxicity (LMC).

Early studies concerned assessment of the ability of BALB/c mice to reject skin allografts across the major (H-2) histocompatability locus (14). For these studies BALB/c (H-2^d) mice were infected with FLV at varying time intervals before grafting with skin from either C₃H (H-2^k) or C57B1/6 (H-2^b) mice. Results of a typical experiment of this type are presented in Table 1.

There was an impaired ability to reject allografts in BALB/c mice infected with FLV 10 days or longer before the receipt of grafts from either C₃H or C57B1/6 mice. No differences in allograft rejection were observed when the duration of infection was less than 10 days. Allograft rejection studies, although generally agreed to be an indicator of a cell-mediated immune function, have several limitations. The ability to determine the mechanism of suppression is hampered by the limited number of manipulations that can be performed on a grafted intact animal. The lack of precision and sensitivity of the method limits its value for study of the early events in leukemogenesis and immune suppression. For these reasons we used the method of macrophage migration inhibition. Studies by Bloom and Bennett revealed that sensitized lymphocytes upon exposure to antigen would release migration inhibitory factor (MIF) (4). For these experiments BALB/c or C57B1/6 mice were sensitized with complete Freund's adjuvant before infection with FLV (19, 20). At varying time intervals after infection, the ability of spleen cells to migrate in the presence or absence of purified protein derivative (PPD) was assayed. The results of one such study are presented in Table 2.

Table 1. Allograft rejection in control and FLV-infected mice

Recipient group[a]	Day of infection in relation to day of grafting	Mean survival time (days) of graft from	
		C57 B1/6	C₃H
Control BALB/c	—	9.3	8.9
FLV-infected BALB/c	−1	8.9	9.1
	−5	8.1	9.7
	−10	14.8	13.5
	−20	>20	>20

[a]Groups of 8–10 young adult (8–12 weeks) BALB/c mice were inoculated i.p. with approximately 500 ID$_{50}$ of FLV on day indicated in relation to day of grafting.

Table 2. Effect of inoculation of FLV on MIF production

Experimental group[a]	% Migration inhibition		
	DBA/2	BALB/c	C57 B1/6
Sensitized, control	48	48	43
Sensitized FLV-1	45	43	36
Sensitized FLV-3	17	21	43
Sensitized FLV-7	15	3	47
Sensitized FLV-10	13	5	53

[a]Groups of mice were sensitized with supplemented complete Freund's adjuvant 21 days before infection with FLV. Mice were infected with FLV at the time indicated before performing the indirect assay to assess the production of MIF.

These results demonstrate a marked reduction in the ability of sensitized lymphocytes from FLV-infected animals to produce MIF in both the susceptible DBA/2 and BALB/c animals. In contrast, the resistant C57B1/6 mice exhibit no appreciable diminution in MIF production following administration of FLV. The FLV-induced defect is in the MIF secreting cell and not in the migrating indicator cell. In spite of its advantages over allograft rejection, the macrophage migration inhibition technique does not differentiate between two possible causes of suppression. The first is that all cells are being suppressed; the second is that a given fraction or proportion of the cells is being completely inhibited while the remainder are producing normal levels of MIF. The experimental technique that appeared capable of resolving this question is the lymphocyte mediated cytotoxicity method (8, 17).

BALB/c mice were sensitized with an alloantigen-bearing lymphoma (EL-4) cell that was maintained by passage in the ascites form in C57B1/6 mice (21). At varying time intervals after sensitization, mice were infected with FLV. At the peak day (day 11) of the immune response, the ability of splenocyte suspensions from control and FLV-infected mice to lyse the target cells was assessed by the release of ^{51}Cr. The cytotoxic potential of splenocytes from control and infected mice are given in Table 3. The efficiency of cytolysis decreases following infection of susceptible BALB/c mice with FLV. No marked depression in cytolytic activity is observed under similar experimental conditions in the resistant C57B1/6 mouse.

The ability of FLV-infected spleen cells to influence the cyto-

Table 3. Cytolytic activity of BALB/c and C57 Bl/6 splenocytes to alloantigen-bearing target cell following administration of FLV

Experimental group[a]	Day FLV administered in relation to day of assay	Cytolytic activity[b] Splenocyte source	
		BALB/c	C57 Bl/6
Control	—	1.00	1.00
FLV-infected	−1	0.62	0.91
	−5	0.22	0.83
	−11	0.01	1.00
	−19	<0.01	0.59

[a]Groups of mice were sensitized by i.p. inoculation of alloantigen-bearing tumor cells 11 days before assay. BALB/c (H-2^d) mice were immunized with the EL-4 lymphoma propagated in C57Bl/6 (H-2^b) mice while C57Bl/6 mice were immunized with the P-815 mastocytoma tumor passaged in DBA/2 (H-2^d) mice. Groups of mice were infected with FLV on the days indicated.

[b]Cytotoxic activity is expressed as the ratio of the number of splenocytes (FLV infected group) required to lyse 10% of the alloantigen-bearing target cells/number of control splenocytes required to lyse 10% of the alloantigen bearing target cells.

toxic potential of sensitized lymphocytes from normal mice has been determined. Splenocytes from normal animals immunized with alloantigen are diluted with splenocytes derived from nonimmunized FLV-infected mice; the results of an experiment of this nature are presented in Table 4. Inhibition in excess of that caused by dilution with normal cells is induced by dilution with spleen cells from FLV-infected animals. Suppression increases as the time interval of infection increases; the degree of suppression also increases as the infecting dose of virus is increased. The suppression in this case might have been caused by a direct effect of the virus on the effector cell population. In order to test this possibility, dilutions of stock virus preparations were incubated with suspensions of splenocytes from normal sensitized animals. These studies demonstrated that the direct addition of infectious FLV into the assay system has no suppressive effect on lymphocyte-mediated cytotoxicity under the experimental conditions employed. Extracts of FLV-infected spleens that were free of infectious virus when incubated with effector cells from normal animals were capable of markedly inhibiting cytotoxic activity. Suppressive activity of the extracts also appears to be a function of the time interval following infection and the infecting

Table 4. Supression of lymphocyte-mediated cytotoxicity by spleen cells from FLV-infected mice

	% of Control[b]	
Experimental group[a]	5×10^6 cells	10×10^6 cells
Control	100	100
FLV, 2 Days	96	90
5 Days	86	81
10 Days	73	50
18 Days	54	27

[a]Groups of mice were infected at the day indicated before the time of assay.
[b]The specific cytolysis observed when 1×10^5 target (EL-4) cells, 5×10^6 splenocytes from immunized mice, and either 5×10^6 or 10×10^6 splenocytes from nonimmunized mice were incubated for 5 hr at 37°C was assigned a value of 100%. The specific cytolysis observed when either 5×10^6 or 10×10^6 splenocytes from FLV-infected, nonimmunized mice were substituted in the reaction mixture is presented as a percent of the control cytolysis.

dose of virus. The active component of the extract of virus infected cells has not yet been isolated or identified. However, suppressive activity is not altered by exposure to DNAse, RNAse, neuraminidase, anti-FLV serum, or 56°C for 30 min. The activity is completely abrogated by incubation with trypsin. Further studies are now in progress to characterize the active protein in the extract as well as to characterize the cell population responsible for the production of the suppressive factor.

III. DISCUSSION

There is a generalized impairment in the ability of FLV-infected mice to function in several correlates of cell-mediated immune function. The early observation that allograft rejection was impaired suggested that a thymus cell function was indeed impaired in FLV-infected mice. The role of these cells in preventing tumor initiation and growth has been considered by a number of investigators as being most important in determining the outcome of the host-tumor interaction (1, 23). In contrast to previous studies on humoral immunity, the allograft studies suggested that suppression of a cell-mediated immune response was a rather late event in leukemogenesis, since prolongation of skin graft survival was noted only at intervals of 10 days or longer after infection (*1*). Graft rejection might be less sensitive to FLV infection or the T cells or other cells participating in the graft rejection may be affected by FLV only late in the disease process.

Studies using the macrophage migration inhibition technique demonstrated a rapid suppression of the production and release of MIF by FLV-infection of susceptible strains of mice. The effect of virus infection is on the lymphocyte component of the reaction and not on the migrating indicator cells. Appropriate controls tend to rule out any contribution of either virus particles or virus-antibody complexes to the observed depression. The production of MIF in the guinea pig is not exclusively a T-cell product since PPD sensitized spleen cell suspensions depleted of T cells can produce MIF as well as lymphotoxin (*5*). As a consequence, the previous interpretation of studies with MMI may require revision if indeed a similar situation prevails in the mouse.

Studies using the lymphocyte-mediated cytotoxicity technique, a T-cell-mediated phenomenon, demonstrate a rapid suppression of cytolytic activity of sensitized cells shortly after infection of susceptible mice with FLV. Such suppression does not appear to be mediated by a direct virus–effector cell interaction. It is possible that spleen cells from FLV-infected mice secrete a "factor" that is capable of inhibiting lymphocyte-mediated cytolysis. The relation of this factor to the suppressor cells observed in normal and virus-infected mice is not known (*15, 18*).

At present it is not known whether this factor is produced by either B cells, T cells, or macrophages, nor whether the virus alters the recognition step or the cytolytic phase of the cytotoxic reaction.

LITERATURE CITED

1. Allison, A. C. and H. Friedman (1970). Immunosuppression and cell mediated immunity in relation to virus infections. *In:* Int. Virol. 2, J. Melnick, Ed., pp. 310–317. S. Karger, New York.
2. Axelrad, A. A. and R. A. Steeves (1964). Assay for Friend leukemia virus: Rapid quantitative method based on enumeration of macroscopic spleen foci in mice. Virology 24:513–518.
3. Bennett, M. and R. A. Steeves (1970). Immunocompetent cell functions in mice infected with Friend leukemia virus. J. Nat. Cancer Inst. 44:1107–1119.
4. Bloom, B. R. and B. Bennett (1971). The assay of inhibition of macrophage migration and the production of MIF and skin reac-

tive factor (SRF). *In:* In Vitro Methods in Cell-Mediated Immunity, B. R. Bloom and P. Glade, Eds., pp. 235–247. Academic Press, New York.

5. Bloom, B. R., G. Stoner, J. Gaffney, E. Shevach, and I. Green (1975). Production of migration inhibitory factor and lymphotoxin by non-T cells. Eur. J. Immunol. 5:218–220.

6. Borella, L. (1971). The immunosuppressive effects of Rauscher leukemia virus upon spleen cells cultured in cell-impermeable diffusion chambers. II. Effects upon IgM and IgG immunologic memory and on the response ot PHA and stimulation with allogeneic cells. J. Immunol. 107:464–475.

7. Ceglowski, W. S., G. U. LaBadie, L. Mills, and H. Friedman (1973). Suppression of the humoral immune response by Friend leukemia virus. *In:* Virus Tumorigenesis and Immunogenesis, W. S. Ceglowski and H. Friedman, Eds., pp. 167–177. Academic Press, New York.

8. Cerottini, J. C., A. A. Nordin, and K. T. Brunner (1970). Specific in vitro cytotoxicity of thymus-derived lymphocytes sensitized to alloantigens. Nature 228:1308–1309.

9. Chirigos, M. A., K. Perk, W. Tumer, B. Burka, and M. Gomez (1968). Increased oncogenicity of the murine sarcoma virus (Moloney) by coinfection with murine leukemic viruses. Cancer Res. 28:1055–1063.

10. Dent, P. B., R. D. A. Peterson, and R. A. Good (1965). A defect in cellular immunity during the incubation period of Gross passage A leukemia in C3H mice. Proc. Soc. Exp. Biol. Med. 119:867–871.

11. Dent, P. B. (1972). Immunodepression by oncogenic viruses. Prog. Med. Virol. 14:1–35.

12. Frey-Wettstein, M. and E. F. Hays (1970). Immune response in preleukemic mice. Infect. Immunity 2:398–403.

13. Friedman, H. and W. S. Ceglowski (1971). Immunosuppression by tumor viruses: Effects of leukemia viruses infection on the immune response. *In:* Progress in Immunology, B. Amos, Ed., pp. 815–830. Academic Press, New York.

14. Friedman, H., H. Melnick, L. Mills, and W. S. Ceglowski (1973). Depressed allograft immunity in leukemia virus infected mice. Transplant Proc. 5:981–988.

15. Gershon, R. K., P. Cohen, R. Hencin, and S. A. Liebhaber (1972). Suppressor T cells. J. Immunol. 108:586–590.

16. Hayry, P., D. Rago, and V. Defendi (1970). Inhibition of PHA and alloantigen induced lymphocyte stimulation by Rauscher leukemia virus. J. Nat. Cancer Inst. 44:1311–1319.

17. Henney, C. S. (1971). Quantitation of the cell-mediated immune response. I. The number of cytolytically active mouse lymphoid cells induced by immunization with allogeneic mastocytoma cells. J. Immunol. 107:1558–1566.

18. Kirchner, H., T. M. Chused, R. B. Herberman, H. T. Holden, and D. H. Lavrin (1974). Evidence of suppressor cell activity in spleens of mice bearing primary tumors induced by Moloney sarcoma virus. J. Exp. Med. 139:1473–1487.

19. Mortensen, R. F., W. S. Ceglowski, and H. Friedman (1973). Leukemia virus-induced immunosuppression. IX. Depression of delayed hypersensitivity and MIF production after infection of mice with Friend leukemia virus. J. Immunol. 111:1810–1819.

20. Mortensen, R. F., W. S. Ceglowski, and H. Friedman (1974). Susceptibility and resistance to Friend leukemia virus: Effect on production of migration-inhibition factor. J. Nat. Cancer Inst. 52:499–505.

21. Mortensen, R. F., W. S. Ceglowski, and H. Friedman (1974). Leukemia virus-induced immunosuppression. X. Depression of T cell-mediated cytotoxicity after infection of mice with Friend leukemia virus. J. Immunol. 112:2077–2086.

22. Notkins, A. L., S. E. Mergenhagen, and R. J. Howard (1970). Effect of virus infections on the function of the immune system. Ann. Rev. Microbiol. 24:525–538.

23. Prehn, R. T. (1969). The relationship of immunology to carcinogenesis. Ann. N. Y. Acad. Sci. 164:499–462.

24. Rowe, W. P., W. E. Pugh, and J. W. Hartley (1970). Plaque assay technique for murine leukemia viruses. Virology 42:1136–1139.

25. Salaman, M. H. (1969). Immunodepression by viruses. Antibiot. Chemother. 15:393–406.

26. Schneider, M. and J. F. Dore (1969). Effect of injection of a leukemogenic virus (Friend) on the immune reactions of mice sensitive and resistant to the virus. Rev. Franc. Clin. Biol. 14:1010–1014.

CHAPTER 9

Immune Activation
of Endogenous Viruses

M. S. Hirsch

I. INTRODUCTION

The interactions between lymphocytes and C-type oncornaviruses are complex and poorly understood. Other chapters in this book review the immunosuppressive properties of murine C-type viruses on humoral and cell-mediated responses (7, 12). Recent studies have shown that murine oncornaviruses can also induce proliferation of autoaggressor lymphocytes (37—39). This review is concerned with the opposite side of this immunologic coin, i.e., the activation of endogenous viruses as a consequence of certain specific lymphocytic responses against antigens or mitogens. Since this phenomenon was first described in 1970 (19), it has been the subject of intensive study in many laboratories (2, 3, 15, 20–24, 29, 33, 35, 36, 40, 42, 47). Both in vivo and in vitro studies are briefly summarized in this review.

II. IN VIVO IMMUNOLOGIC
ACTIVATION OF ENDOGENOUS VIRUSES

A. Graft-versus-host Reactions (GVHR)

When parental murine lymphoid cells are inoculated into F_1 hybrid mice, graft-versus-host reactions (GVHR) may result from responses

Work from our laboratory described in this review was supported by United States Public Health Service Grant 12464-04 and by Contract NIH 72-2012 within the Virus Cancer Program of the National Cancer Institute.

of donor lymphocytes against histocompatibility-associated antigens derived from the opposite parent. Depending on the strains involved and the ages of the recipients, a variety of immunopathologic syndromes have been observed (3, 10, 20). Our studies have been largely concerned with one particular strain combination. When BALB/c splenocytes are injected intraperitoneally into 6–10-week-old (BALB/c $\times$ A/J)F$_1$ mice, the recipients develop malignant lymphomas, particularly reticulum cell sarcomas, at a markedly increased rate when compared with uninjected littermates (3). The tumors in the (BALB/c $\times$ A/J)F$_1$ recipients are predominantly of recipient origin (14). We have shown that following injection of parental cells, C-type viruses can be detected in spleens from the majority of recipient mice, whereas they are rarely detected in uninjected F$_1$ mice or in donor BALB/c mice at this age (19). Treatment of donor cells with mitomycin C or anti-θ serum prevents both GVHR and virus activation from occurring. These observations have been confirmed and extended in other laboratories (4, 35, 36, 40), and several facts appear clear. Following GVHR, both ecotropic and xenotropic virus can be activated (4, 20, 40). Reactions against certain other antigen complexes, e.g., sheep erythrocytes or Freund's adjuvant, do not result in comparable degrees of virus activation. Cell-free extracts of spleens from GVHR mice that contain ecotropic viruses are oncogenic for newborn F$_1$ mice and induce the same type of reticulum cell sarcomas as seen in the GVHR animal (4). During GVHR and virus activation, a variable degree of immunosuppression is observed (35, 36, 42). What remains unclear is whether such animals are hyporesponsive to their own activated viruses and whether this hyporesponsiveness contributes to virus replication, persistence, and neoplasia. It cannot be said with certainty that the activated viruses are causally related to the tumors that develop in the GVHR animals, although usually acceptable standards, i.e., Koch's postulates, have been fulfilled. It can also not be said with certainty that what has been called virus activation may not be amplification of subthreshold levels of infectious virus in a host that is immunologically altered by a GVHR. I am not sure that either of these questions can be answered with presently available techniques. Nevertheless, the most reasonable interpretation of the accumulated data would appear to be that following induction of a GVHR, C-type viruses are activated from responding T cells; these agents subsequently infect host reticulum cells and alter them in such a way as to result in their unrestricted proliferation culminating in malignancy.

B.   Skin Graft Rejection Reactions

The placement of allogeneic skin grafts onto BALB/c mice also elicits an immune response against foreign histocompatibility antigens. If the grafts are rapidly rejected, the response is transient. If certain immunosuppressive therapy is given to the graft recipient, graft maintenance is prolonged. We have found that the latter situation is highly conducive to the activation of C-type viruses (21, 24). Both mice sharing the same H-2 locus with BALB/c recipients (DBA/2) or differing at this locus (A/J) have been used as skin graft donors, with comparable results. Immunosuppressive regimens have consisted of varying doses of antilymphocytic serum (ALS), cyclophosphamide, or cortisone. As shown in Table 1, regimens that result in significant graft prolongation (either high-dose ALS or high-dose cyclophosphamide) lead to high incidences of virus activation, whereas regimens that do not prolong graft maintenance do not lead to virus activation. The viruses activated from some grafted animals are ecotropic and from others xenotropic; occasional animals have both types of virus. At least some of the activated ecotropic C-type viruses are oncogenic, inducing thymic lymphomas when inoculated into newborn NIH-Swiss mice. A kinetic study of virus activation following skin grafting indicates that viruses are first detectable 1–2 weeks following graft placement in draining regional nodes; thereafter, maximum virus titers are achieved in the spleen (24). Viruses were not detected at skin graft sites, thymuses, or tails of recipient animals, and were never found in donor grafts. The circumstantial evidence thus indicates that endogenous viruses are activated from responding lymphoid cells of recipient animals, and that the replication of these viruses is then amplified by concomitant immunosuppression.

Histological changes observed in spleens of mice receiving skin grafts and either high-dose ALS or high-dose cyclophosphamide are remarkably similar to those seen in mice with GVHR (24). At times when C-type viruses are first detectable, depletion of small lymphocytes in periarteriolar areas is apparent, and hyperplasia of large reticular cells and granulocyte precursors is marked.

C-type viruses are apparently not the only murine viruses that

Table 1. Activation of viruses following skin grafting and various immunosuppressive regimens

Group	Number of mice	Skin graft[a]	Suppressive treatment	Skin-graft MST ± SE (days)	Mean spleen weight ± SE (g)	Number of virus-positive mice			
						Mouse-tropic	Xeno-tropic	Mouse-tropic + xeno-tropic	Total
A	15	+	None	14.8±2.1	0.157±0.013	2	0	0	2(13%)
B	20	+	ALS	28	0.232±0.016[b]	4	5	4	13(65%)[c]
C	13	+	High-dose cyclophosphamide	20.8±5.8	0.209±0.018[d]	6	1	2	9(69%)[c]
D	16	+	Low-dose cyclophosphamide	16.0±5.8	0.189±0.020	0	0	0	0(0%)
E	14	+	High-dose cortisone	15.9±4.1	0.086±0.007[b]	0	1	0	1(7%)
F	18	+	Low-dose cortisone	15.1±1.8	0.127±0.004[d]	0	0	0	0(0%)
G	15	−	High-dose cyclophosphamide	—	0.118±0.010	0	0	0	0(0%)
H	15	−	None	—	0.124±0.012	0	0	0	0(0%)

[a]BALB/c mice grafted with DBA/2 skin.
[b]$p < 0.01$ compared with Group A (t-test).
[c]$p < 0.01$ compared with Group A (Chi-square).
[d]$p < 0.05$ compared with Group A (t-test).

may be activated by host-versus-graft reactions in vivo. Wu et al. have recently reported that latent murine cytomegalovirus (CMV) can be activated in spleens of C_3H/He mice engrafted with either skin or lymphoid cells from a variety of different mouse strains (47). It is thus likely that the in vivo immunologic activation phenomenon will be extended to other murine viruses that are latent in lymphocytes, and also that it will not be restricted to mice,

A summary of in vivo virus activation studies is shown in Table 2 but will be demonstrated in other species as well.

III. IN VITRO ACTIVATION OF VIRUSES FROM LYMPHOCYTES

A. Mixed Lymphocyte Reactions (MLR)

Considerable effort has been devoted toward activating C-type viruses from fibroblasts in vitro using a variety of inducing agents including halogenated pyrimidines, hormones, and x-irradiation (17, 46). These studies have now been extended to a variety of species other than mouse (17). In 1972, it was shown that endogenous C-type viruses could also be activated from lymphocytes by a mixed lymphocyte reaction between BALB/c and (BALB/c $\times$ A/J)F_1 spleen cells (20). As with the GVHR in vivo, this MLR primarily represents BALB/c T lymphocytes reacting against A/J histocompatibility-related antigens. The viruses detected were observed by electron microscopy budding exclusively from lymphoblasts (2), suggesting that responding BALB/c cells are the source of the virus. The frequency of virus positivity is less, and the titers of virus obtained are lower in the MLR than in the GVHR. However,

Table 2. Activation of viruses during in vivo lymphocytic responses

Response	C-type		CMV
	Ecotropic	Xenotropic	
GVHR	+	+	NT[a]
Skin transplantation	+	+	+
Sheep red blood cells	—	NT	NT
Freund's adjuvant	—	NT	NT
Allogeneic splenocytes	—	NT	NT

[a]Not tested.

both types of reactions are associated with the activation of ecotropic and xenotropic C-type viruses (20, 41).

Latent CMV has also been activated from murine lymphocytes in vitro by reactivity against allogeneic but not syngeneic fibroblasts (33). The activation of CMV was presumably secondary to reactivity against histocompatibility-related antigens, although the cells from which virus was obtained appeared to be B, rather than T, lymphocytes. As in the in vivo activation of endogenous viruses, it is unlikely that in vitro immunologic activation will be limited to C-type oncornaviruses and CMV, or to the murine species. Studies are currently underway in several laboratories to evaluate the possibility that latent human viruses may be activated by immunological means.

B. Mitogens

Murine lymphocytes have been treated with a variety of specific antigens and nonspecific mitogens (Table 3), in an attempt to activate C-type viruses by means other than histocompatibility-related reactions (15, 20, 30, 36). Until recently, these attempts have been unsuccessful. However, it has now been shown that bacterial lipopolysaccharide (LPS), a B-lymphocyte mitogen, is a specific and efficient inducer of a particular class of xenotropic BALB/c C-type viruses (15, 30). Concanavalin A (Con A) could also induce xenotropic viruses from lymphocytes, although it was a less efficient inducer than LPS (15, 30); in one study, Con A required the additional inducing effect of a halogenated pyrimidine,

Table 3. Activation of viruses during in vitro lymphocytic responses

Agent or response	C-type		CMV
	Ecotropic	Xenotropic	
Histocompatibility antigens	+	+	+
IUDR or BUDR	+	+	NT[a]
Prolonged culture	+	NT	NT
Lipopolysaccharide	−	+	+
Concanavalin A	−	+	−
Phytohemagglutinin	−	−	−
Pokeweed mitogen	−	NT	−
Antilymphocyte serum	−	NT	NT
Sheep red blood cells	−	NT	NT

[a]Not tested.

5-bromo-2'-deoxyuridine (BUDR), for viral activation (*30*); similarly the activating effects of LPS were potentiated by subsequent addition of BUDR. Halogenated pyrimidines by themselves can also induce C-type viruses from lymphocytes and fibroblasts, presumably by a mechanism other than stimulation of lymphocyte proliferation (*30, 36*). Neither LPS nor Con A was capable of inducing virus from fibroblasts (*15*), and phytohemagglutinin (PHA) has not been reported to induce C-type viruses from either lymphocytes or fibroblasts. Thus, there remains some degree of specificity among mitogens in their capacity to activate C-type viruses. Although lymphocyte blastogenesis may be a prerequisite for mitogenic or antigenic activation of viruses, this alone is not sufficient. The selection of certain subpopulations of lymphocytes for stimulation may be a more important factor in determining if viruses are activated, and which classes of viruses are produced. Presently, it appears that certain T-lymphocytes may be stimulated during MLR to produce either ecotropic or xenotropic viruses, whereas B-lymphocytes may produce xenotropic viruses after appropriate mitogenic stimulation.

Culture of murine lymphocytes in vitro regularly leads to the spontaneous expression of certain C-type viral proteins (*27*), and occasionally leads to the production of infectious C-type viruses. This may represent release from in vivo immunologic restraints to virus production, analogous to the pattern observed when Burkitt lymphoma cells are cultured in vitro followed by expression of latent Epstein-Barr viruses (*26*). Similar patterns have also been observed with other viruses latent in lymphocytes (*9*).

Mitogenic activation of viruses is not limited to C-type agents. Murine CMV has been activated in vitro from splenic lymphocytes by exposure to the B-cell mitogen, LPS, but not by exposure to PHA, Con A, or pokeweed mitogen (*33*). All mitogens used induced comparable lymphocyte blastogenesis; however, only LPS, in its most mitogenic dose, activated virus. These findings suggest that although lymphocyte proliferation may be a prerequisite for CMV production, activation may be restricted to certain lymphocyte subpopulations.

IV. DISCUSSION

The evidence is now abundant that certain proliferative responses of murine lymphocytes can result in the activation or amplification of undetectable endogenous viruses. The important biomedical questions that remain are: (1) Do these observations have relevance to human disease, particularly lymphomagenesis? (2) If so, can the sequence of reactions proceeding from immune reactions to virus activation to cancer be interrupted? To the former question, I can only speculate by analogy. It is now well established that human renal transplant recipients have a markedly increased incidence of viral infections compared to control populations, with members of the herpesvirus group (particularly cytomegalovirus) and members of the papovavirus group predominating (8, 11, 28, 43, 54). These patients have also an incidence of lymphoreticular neoplasms, particularly reticulum cell sarcomas, several hundredfold the number that is found in control populations (25, 34). Bone marrow transplant recipients are frequently subject to development of GVHR and also have an unusual propensity towards developing significant cytomegalovirus infections (31, 32); the likelihood of subsequent malignancy in this bone marrow recipient group has not yet been established. Whether transplant recipient populations also have a high incidence of C-type oncornavirus expression has not yet been determined, although techniques for detection of primate C-type viruses have recently been described (13, 41, 44). It appears likely that in both the renal and bone marrow transplant recipient, the combination of chronic histoincompatibility reactions and chronic immunosuppression results in expression of latent endogenous viruses that may or may not be related to subsequent neoplasia.

How such activated endogenous viruses may lead to lymphomas in mouse or man is unclear. Experimental evidence indicates that lymphocytes in certain stages of differentiation may be uniquely susceptible to infection, and infection at these stages may lead to unrestricted lymphoid cell proliferation, culminating in malignancy (18). Loss of feedback control under these circumstances may be due to depletion of "suppressor" T cells (1, 5, 18, 29) or to auto-aggressive elimination of host antivirus or antitumor cells (18, 37–39).

Can the chain from immune activation of viruses to neoplasia be broken? Animal data suggests that it can (22). Interferon has been shown in mice to have both potent antiviral and weak immuno-suppressive effects (6, 22, 23). In the GVHR model, interferon administration can reduce the histocompatibility reaction, diminish C-type virus activation, and prevent lymphoma development (22).

It is hoped that since high titered human interferon preparations are now available for clinical trials, similar studies can be undertaken in human transplant recipients. The transplant recipient may not be the only type of patient susceptible to the immunological activation of viruses. A great many chronic diseases are associated with persistent antigenic challenge and the chronic presence of indigenous or iatrogenic immunosuppression. Many of these disorders, e.g., Sjögren's syndrome and ulcerative colitis, also have an increased incidence of tumors. In future years, the search for viruses in such disorders should perhaps be directed towards the responding lymphocytes rather than the antigenic target cells.

LITERATURE CITED

1. Allison, A. C. (1973). Mechanisms of tolerance and autoimmunity. Ann. Rheum. Dis 32:283–293.
2. André-Schwartz, J., R. S. Schwartz, M. S. Hirsch, S. M. Phillips, and P. H. Black (1973). Activation of leukemia viruses by graft-versus-host and mixed-lymphocyte culture reactions: electron microscopic evidence of C-type particles. J. Nat. Cancer Inst. 51:507–518.
3. Armstrong, M. Y. K., E. Gleichmann, H. Gleichmann, L. Beldotti, J. André-Schwartz, and R. S. Schwartz (1970). Chronic allogeneic disease. II. Development of lymphomas. J. Exp. Med. 132:417–439.
4. Armstrong, M. Y. K., N. H. Ruddle, M. B. Lipman, and F. F. Richards (1973). Tumor induction by immunologically activated murine leukemia virus. J. Exp. Med. 137:1163–1179.
5. Barthold, D. R., S. Kysela, and A. D. Steinberg (1974). Decline in suppressor T cell function with age in female NZB mice. J. Immunol. 112:9–16.
6. Brodeur, B. R. and T. C. Merigan (1974). Suppressive effect of interferon on the humoral immune response to sheep red blood cells in mice. J. Immunol. 113:1319–1325.
7. Ceglowski, W. S. (1975). Effects of leukemia viruses on cell-mediated immune responses, this volume, p. 165.
8. Coleman, D. V., S. D. Gardner, and A. M. Field (1973). Human polyomavirus infection in renal allograft recipients. Br. Med. J. 3:371–375.
9. Deinhardt, F. (1973). Herpesvirus saimiri. In: The Herpesviruses, A. S. Kaplan, Ed., pp. 595–625. Academic Press, New York.
10. Elkins, W. L. (1971). Cellular immunology and the pathogenesis of graft versus host reactions. Prog. Allergy 15:78–187.
11. Fiala, M., J. E. Payne, T. V. Berne, T. C. Moore, W. Henle, J. Z. Montgomerie, S. N. Chatterjee, and L. B. Guze (1975). Epidem-

iology of cytomegalovirus infection following transplantation and immunosuppression. J. Inf. Dis. 132:421–433.

12. Friedman, H. (1975). Impairment of antibody forming mechanisms by leukemia viruses, this volume, p. 215.

13. Gallagher, R. E. and R. C. Gallo (1975). Type C RNA tumor virus isolated from cultured human acute myelogeneous leukemia cells. Science 187:350–353.

14. Gleichmann, E., H. Gleichmann, R. S. Schwartz, A. Weinblatt, and M. Y. K. Armstrong (1975). Immunologic induction of malignant lymphoma: identification of donor and host tumors in the graft-versus-host-model. J. Nat. Cancer Inst. 54:107–116.

15. Greenberger, J. S., S. M. Phillips, J. R. Stephenson, and S. A. Aaronson (1975). Induction of type-C RNA virus by lipopolysaccharide. J. Immunol. 115:317–320.

16. Herberman, R. B. (1975). Cell-mediated immunity in murine virus tumor systems, this volume, p. xxx.

17. Hirsch, M. S. and P. H. Black (1974). Activation of mammalian leukemia viruses. Adv. Virus Res. 19:265–313.

18. Hirsch, M. S. and M. R. Proffitt (1975). Viruses and autoimmunity. In: Viral Immunology and Immunopathology, A. Notkins, Ed. Academic Press, New York.

19. Hirsch, M. S., P. H. Black, G. S. Tracy, S. Leibowitz, and R. S. Schwartz (1970). Leukemia virus activation in chronic allogeneic disease. Proc. Nat. Acad. Sci. U.S.A. 67:1914–1917.

20. Hirsch, M. S., S. M. Phillips, C. Solnik, P. H. Black, R. S. Schwartz, and C. B. Carpenter (1972). Activation of leukemia viruses by graft-versus-host and mixed lymphocyte reactions in vitro. Proc. Nat. Acad. Sci. U.S.A. 69:1069–1072.

21. Hirsch, M. S., D. A. Ellis, P. H. Black, A. P. Monaco, and M. L. Wood (1973). Leukemia virus activation during homograft rejection. Science 180:500–502.

22. Hirsch, M. S., D. A. Ellis, M. R. Proffitt, P. H. Black, and M. A. Chirigos (1973). Effects of interferon on leukemia virus activation in graft versus host disease. Nature New Biol. 244:102–103.

23. Hirsch, M. S., D. A. Ellis, P. H. Black, A. P. Monaco, and M. L. Wood (1974). Immunosuppressive effects of an interferon preparation in vivo. Transplantation 17:234–236.

24. Hirsch, M. S., D. A. Ellis, A. P. Kelly, M. R. Proffitt, P. H. Black, A. P. Monaco, and M. L. Wood (1975). Activation of C-type viruses during skin graft rejection of the mouse. Interrelationships between immunostimulation and immunosuppression. Int. J. Cancer 15:493–502.

25. Hoover, R. and J. F. Fraumeni, Jr. (1973). Risk of cancer in renal-transplant recipients. Lancet ii:55–57.

26. Klein, G. 1973. The Epstein-Barr virus. In: The Herpesviruses, A. S. Kaplan, Ed., pp. 521–555. Academic Press, New York.

27. Lonai, P., A. Declève, and H. S. Kaplan (1974). Spontaneous induction of endogenous murine leukemia virus-related antigen expres-

sion during short-term in vitro incubation of mouse lymphocytes. Proc. Nat. Acad. Sci. U.S.A. 71:2008–2012.

28. Lopez, C., R. L. Simmons, S. M. Mauer, J. S. Najarian, and R. A. Good (1974). Association of renal allograft rejection with virus infections. Am. J. Med. 56:280–289.

29. Melief, C. J. M., S. Datta, S. Louie, and R. S. Schwartz (1974). Immunologic activation of murine leukemia viruses. Cancer 34:1481–1487.

30. Moroni, C., G. Schumann, M. Robert-Guroff, E. R. Suter, and D. Martin (1975). Induction of endogenous murine C-type virus in spleen cell cultures treated with mitogens and 5-bromo-2'-deoxyuridine. Proc. Nat. Acad. Sci. U.S.A. 72:535–538.

31. Myers, J. D., H. C. Spencer, Jr., J. C. Watts, M. B. Gregg, J. A. Stewart, R. H. Troupin, and E. D. Thomas (1975). Cytomegalovirus pneumonia after human marrow transplantation. Ann. Int. Med. 82:181–188.

32. Neiman, P., P. B. Wasserman, B. B. Wentworth, G. F. Kau, K. G. Lerner, R. Storb, C. D. Buckner, R. A. Clift, A. Fefer, L. Fass, H. Glucksberg, and E. D. Thomas (1973). Interstitial pneumonia and cytomegalovirus infection as complications of human marrow transplantation. Transplantation 15:478–485.

33. Olding, L. B., F. C. Jensen, and M. B. A. Oldstone (1975). Pathogenesis of cytomegalovirus infection. I. Activation of virus from bone marrow-derived lymphocytes by in vitro allogenic reaction. J. Exp. Med. 141:561–572.

34. Penn, I. and T. E. Starzl (1972). Malignant tumors arising de novo in immunosuppressed organ transplant recipients. Transplantation 14:407–417.

35. Phillips, S. M., H. Gleichmann, M. S. Hirsch, P. H. Black, J. P. Merrill, R. S. Schwartz, and C. B. Carpenter (1975). Cellular immunity in the mouse. IV. Altered thymic dependent lymphocyte reactivity in the chronic graft versus host reaction and leukemia virus activation. Cell. Immunol. 15:152–168.

36. Phillips, S. M., M. S. Hirsch, J. André-Schwartz, C. Solnik, P. Black, R. S. Schwartz, J. P. Merrill, and C. B. Carpenter (1975). Cellular immunity in the mouse. V. Further studies on leukemia virus activation in allogeneic reactions of mice: stimulatory parameters. Cell. Immunol. 15:169–179.

37. Proffitt, M. R., M. S. Hirsch, and P. H. Black (1973). Murine leukemia: a virus-induced autoimmune disease? Science 182:821–823.

38. Proffitt, M. R., M. S. Hirsch, B. Gheridian, I. F. C. McKenzie, and P. H. Black (1975). Immunological mechanisms in the pathogenesis of virus-induced murine leukemia. I. Autoreactivity. Int. J. Cancer 15:221–229.

39. Proffitt, M. R., M. S. Hirsch, I. F. C. McKenzie, B. Gheridian, and P. H. Black (1975). Immunological mechanisms in the pathogenesis of virus-induced murine leukemia II. Characterization of autoreactive thymocytes. Int. J. Cancer 15:230–240.

40. Sherr, C. J., M. M. Lieber, and G. J. Todaro (1974). Mixed spleno-cyte cultures and graft versus host reactions selectively induce an "S-tropic" murine type-C virus. Cell 1:55–58.
41. Sherr, C. J. and G. J. Todaro (1974). Type C viral antigens in man. I. Antigens related to endogenous primate virus in human tumors. Proc. Nat. Acad. Sci. U.S.A. 71:4703–4707.
42. Solnik, C., H. Gleichmann, M. Kavanah, and R. S. Schwartz (1973). Immunosuppression and malignant lymphomas in graft versus host reactions. Cancer Res. 33:2068–2077.
43. Spencer, E. S. and H. K. Anderson (1970). Clinically evident, non-terminal infections with herpesviruses and the wart virus in im-munosuppressed renal allograft recipients. Br. Med. J. 3:251–254.
44. Strand, M. and J. T. August (1974). Type C RNA virus gene ex-pression in human tissue. J. Virol. 14:1584–1596.
45. Strauch, B., L. Andrews, N. Siegel, and G. Miller. (1974). Oro-pharyngeal excretion of Epstein-Barr virus by renal transplant recipients and other patients treated with immunosuppressive drugs. Lancet 1:234–237.
46. Todaro, G. J. and R. J. Huebner (1972). The viral oncogene hyp-othesis: new evidence. Proc. Nat. Acad. Sci. U.S.A. 69:1009–1015.
47. Wu, B. C., J. N. Dowling, J. A. Armstrong, and M. Ho (1975). Activation of chronic murine cytomegalovirus in C_3H/He mouse by allograft. Amer. Soc. Microbiol. Proc. (abstract) p. 273.

CHAPTER 10

Do Intracisternal Type A Particles From Plasmacytoma Have Immunosuppressive Activity?

D. Giacomoni, J. Katzmann,
S. Chandra, and P. Heller

I. INTRODUCTION

Oncogenic viruses and particularly the leukemogenic viruses cause depression of the immune response in mice. The effect on the immune response varies among these viruses, but they primarily influence immunologic factors that depend on both B cells and T cells. The effect of oncogenic viruses on the host immune mechanisms has been reviewed recently (6). Evidence indicates that leukemia viruses impair the primary and the secondary response to a variety of antigens (2, 18) and that cell-mediated immunity is also impaired (2–4, 7, 16, 19).

Immunodeficiency caused by oncogenic viruses may be a necessary antecedent to the growth of a tumor. Strains of mice resistant to Friend leukemia viruses do not show immunosuppression when infected with the virus (9, 17, 19, 21). It has been shown that immunosuppression stimulates oncogenesis by murine sarcoma virus

This research was supported by a grant from the Chicago Leukemia Research Foundation and from the Veterans Administration Research Fund.

(24). Also, chickens that eventually die of leukosis have significant depression of antibody responses (5).

Impairment of the primary but not of the secondary immunologic response is also observed in BALB/c mice with plasmacytoma (8). The immunosuppression of plasmacytomatous mice has been attributed to a humoral factor (20). The possibility that this factor is released from the plasmacytoma cells and its activity is due to a RNA molecule is suggested by the observation that impairment of primary immunologic response can result from intraperitoneal injection of RNA extracted from plasmacytoma or from plasma of plasmacytomatous mice (22). No immunodeficiency is elicited when RNA from normal spleen or liver is injected into mice or when plasmacytoma RNA is degraded with RNase before injection (22). The following data show that immunodepression can be induced by a subcellular fraction enriched in type A particles and particularly by the RNA extracted from this fraction. Since no plasmacytoma subcellular fraction has been shown to cause malignancy, this system allows the study of tumor-induced immunodeficiency independent of tumor growth.

II. EXPERIMENTAL DATA

The immunosuppressive activity of subcellular fractions from plasmacytoma was determined. Cells of the MOPC 300 tumor were fractionated following the first fractionation steps described by Kuff et al. (13), and the fractions were monitored by electron microscopy (Figure 1). The different fractions obtained were (a) the nuclei, (b) supernatant A (enriched in nonmembrane-bound polysomes), (c) precipitate B (enriched in intracisternal type A particles but containing also reticular membranes, and a few polysomes), and (d) precipitate C (containing most membrane-bound polysomes released by the detergent treatment). Different amounts of these subcellular fractions were injected intraperitoneally into normal mice. Three days later (the time interval that gave optimal immunosuppression when plasmacytoma RNA was used), the mice received 0.3 ml of a 10% suspension of sheep red blood cells (SRBC) intraperitoneally (22). Five days after the injection of SRBC the animals were sacrificed, and the spleen cells were tested in a hemolytic plaque assay (12). Control animals received only SRBC. When amounts of each fraction containing 500 μg of nucleic acids were used, only precipitate B caused a diminution of plaque forming cells by approximately 35% (Table 1, experiment 1). When double amounts of each fraction were used, the highest degree of immunosuppression (70%) was again found in mice injected with precipitate B (Table 1, experiment 2). Nuclei never caused immunosuppression (Table 1). When corresponding subcellular fractions obtained from normal liver were used, no immunosuppression was detected (data not shown).

The data presented in Table 1 suggest that the immunosuppressive activity might be due to the intracisternal type A particles concentrated in precipitate B. Intracisternal type A particles were purified (Figure 2) from MOPC 300, MOPC 104E, and J606 tumors. The immunosuppressive activity of each preparation of type A particles was assessed by the experimental protocol described above. All of them cause immunosuppression (30–50%) in mice compared to control mice injected with "precipitate B" from normal liver and spleen (Table 2, experiment 2). In another experiment (Table 2, experiment 1) type A particles or supernatant A from MOPC 300 were injected into two sets of mice. As expected, mice injected with supernatant A (250 μg) show little inhibition (25%) of their primary immune response to SRBC while a smaller amount (75 μg) of type A particles causes a marked decrease in the immune response (50%).

RNA was extracted from type A particle-rich fractions (precipitate B) and from purified type A particles and the immunosuppressive effect of these RNA preparations was tested. Table 3 shows

Table 1. Immunosuppressive activity of plasmacytoma subcellular fractions[a]

Fraction	Experiment 1 (500 μg)		Experiment 2 (1,000 μg)	
	PFU/10^6 cells	%	PFU/10^6	%
Control (MEM)	930 ± 150	100	780 ± 80	100
Nuclei	950 ± 300	102	600 ± 110	85
A[b]	730 ± 200	80	320 ± 160	41
B[c]	600 ± 100	65	230 ± 80	29
C[d]	820 ± 150	88	400 ± 120	51

[a]Each fraction was injected into five mice 3 days before challenge with SRBC.

[b]Enriched in non-membrane-bound polysomes.

[c]Enriched in type A particles.

[d]Enriched in membrane-bound polysomes.

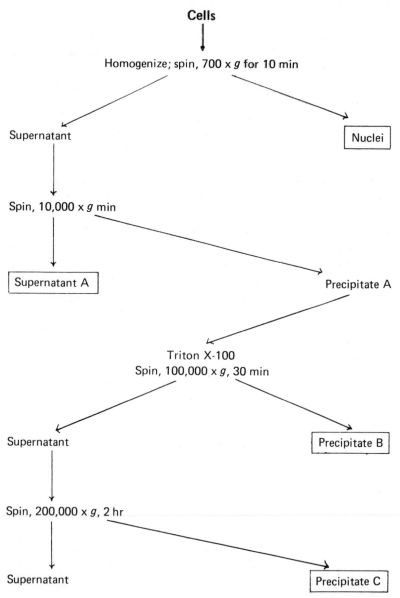

Figure 1. Fractionation of cells. Cells were homogenized at 0°C in 4 volumes of solution A (0.25 M sucrose, 0.05 M Tris, pH 7.6, 0.025 M KCl, and 0.005 M MgCl₂). Nuclei were further purified by washing in solution A containing 0.1% Triton X-100. Precipitate A was resuspended in solution A to a final

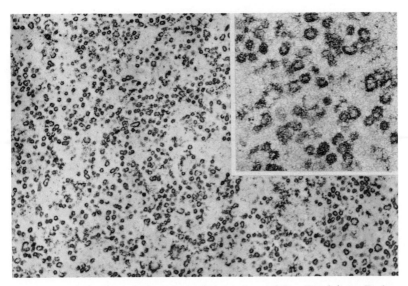

Figure 2. Purification of intracisternal type A particles. Precipitate B (see Figure 1) was suspended in 25% sucrose in 0.05 M sodium citrate pH 7.2, layered over a cushion of 48% sucrose in the same buffer, and spun overnight at 25,000 rpm in a Spinco SW 41 rotor. The pellet at the bottom of the tube was resuspended in 0.05 M sodium citrate, pH 7.2 and layered on top of a sucrose gradient (33–68% w/v) in the same buffer. After 4 hr centrifugation at 40,000 rpm (SW 41) the fractions containing type A particles were collected by centrifugation. For electron microscopy the pellets were fixed overnight in 2.5% glutaraldehyde and then in chrome-osmium for 1 hr, dehydrated in graded concentrations of ethanol, and embedded in Epon-Araldite mixtures. Thin sections cut on LKB-Ultrotome and picked on uncoated grids were stained with lead citrate and uranyl acetate and examined in a Siemens Elmiskop I electron microscope. Insert shows type A particles at a higher magnification; loss of structural integrity of the particles could be due to detergent treatment. × 10,725 (insert × 32,500).

the results of two typical experiments when RNA from the fraction rich in type A particles (precipitate B) was used. In one experiment 100 μg of RNA from precipitate B (see Figure 1) from MOPC 300 tumor caused an 80% decrease in the primary immune response to SRBC when compared with control animals that had received

volume equivalent to half the original weight of the tumor, Triton X-100 was added to a final concentration of 0.4%, and the suspension was forced 5 times through a G23 needle and then diluted with 7 volumes of 0.15 M sodium citrate, pH 7.2 before centrifugation to obtain precipitate B and precipitate C.

192   Giacomoni et al.

Table 2. Immunosuppressive activity of intracisternal type A particles

Fraction	Amount injected (μg)	PFU/10^6 cells	%
Experiment 1[a]			
Control (MEM)	—	295 ± 50	100
Sup. A[b]	250	220 ± 80	75, $p < 0.1$
MOPC 300, A particle	75	140 ± 50	48, $p < 0.001$
Experiment 2[a]			
Control[c]	140	1,700 ± 250	100
MOPC 300, A particle	125	1,050 ± 30	60, $p < 0.05$
MOPC 104E, A particle	125	900 ± 120	50, $p < 0.001$
J606, A particle	100	1,200 ± 200	70, $p < 0.05$

[a]Each fraction was injected into four mice 3 days before challenge with SRBC.
[b]Tumor fraction enriched in non-membrane-bound polysomes.
[c]"Precipitate B" from normal liver and spleen.

Table 3. Immunosuppressive activity of RNA derived from plasmacytoma fractions enriched in type A particles

Fraction	Amount injected (μg)	PFU/10^6 cells	%
Experiment 1[a]			
Mouse liver RNA	200	200 ± 80	100
MOPC 300 "ppt B" RNA	100	40 ± 15	20, $p < 0.001$
Experiment 2[a]			
Saline (control)	—	820 ± 300	100
Mouse liver RNA	300	790 ± 400	96
MOPC 104E "ppt B" RNA	70	60 ± 40	7, $p < 0.001$
MOPC 300 RNA[b]	300	80 ± 60	10, $p < 0.001$

[a]Each RNA preparation was injected into five mice 3 days before challenge with SRBC.
[b]From the unfractionated tumor.

a higher dose (200 μg) of normal liver RNA (Table 3, experiment 1). In another experiment, mouse liver RNA (300 μg per mouse) failed to cause immunodeficiency while a lower dose (70 μg) of RNA from precipitate B of MOPC 104E tumor cells caused a 90% decrease in the number of cells producing antibodies to SRBC (Table 3, experiment 2). RNA from unfractionated MOPC 300 tumor cells (300 μg per mouse) also caused immunodeficiency (90%). In two experiments in which four to five mice received only 20–70 μg of RNA from type A particles of MOPC 300 tumor, the immune response to SRBC was markedly decreased (80–95%) when compared to the immune response of animals that had received higher doses (60–100 μg) of normal mouse liver RNA (Table 4, experiments 1 and 2).

III. DISCUSSION

It can be seen from the experiments reported above that there is great variation in the primary immune response to SRBC from one experiment to another (see, for example, Table 3, experiment 1 versus experiment 2). Within each experiment, however, the immune response was reduced by type A particles, fractions enriched in type A particles, and their RNAs. Precipitate B (corresponding to 500–1000 μg of RNA) decreases the immune response 35–70%. Smaller doses of type A particles (100 μg of RNA) are sufficient to obtain a similar effect, indicating a correlation between immuno-

Table 4. Immunosuppressive activity of RNA isolated from intracisternal type A particles

RNA fraction	Amount injected (μg)	PFU/10^6 cells	%
Experiment 1			
Mouse liver	60	1057 ± 700	100
MOPC 300, A particle	70	194 ± 120	18, $p < 0.001$
Experiment 2			
Mouse liver	100	742 ± 150	100
MOPC 300, A particle	20	39 ± 13	5, $p < 0.001$

suppressive activity and type A particles. Plasmacytoma fractions enriched in free and membrane-bound polysomes and almost devoid of type A particles (supernatant A and precipitate C, respectively, Table 1) possess a minor immunosuppressive activity that we tentatively attribute to either contaminating type A particles or to type A particle specific macromolecules present in these preparations. Nuclei from plasmacytoma cells and subcellular fractions from normal liver have no effect on the immune response. RNA from plasmacytoma, from precipitate B (enriched in type A particles), and from intracisternal type A particles diminish the immune response to SRBC by 80–90%. RNA from type A particles is effective at lower concentrations than is RNA from unfractionated plasmacytoma or from precipitate B, indicating a correlation between type A particle RNA and immunosuppressive activity.

These data suggest that intracisternal type A particles cause immunodeficiency and that their immunosuppressive activity is due to the RNA moiety. We have consistently observed that type A particles yield less reproducible results and never achieve the degree of immunosuppression that is observed when their RNA is used. Since the immunodeficiency in plasmacytomatous mice has been attributed to a humoral factor and to RNA extracted from the plasma of tumor-bearing animals, it will be interesting to isolate this humoral factor and determine its relationship to intracisternal type A particles (20, 22).

Another phenomenon that accompanies the growth of murine and human myeloma is the appearance on the surface of lymphocytes of new immunoglobulins (Ig) with the idiotypic specificity of the myeloma protein (cell conversion (1, 11, 15, 23)). The subcellular localization and some physicochemical characteristics of plasmacytoma RNA that, in vitro and in vivo, can cause cell conversion have been determined (10, 14). The subcellular fractions that caused cell conversion are the same that cause immunodeficiency. Therefore, it is conceivable that during the growth of plasmacytoma, the tumor cells release an RNA-containing particle (related to intracisternal type A particles) that can enter the lymphocytes and change their surface Ig, thus disabling these lymphocytes as antigen receptors and eliciting immunodeficiency. It is conceivable that the subsequent immunodeficiency also lowers the ability of the organism to reject the tumor.

LITERATURE CITED

1. Abdou, N. I. and N. L. Abdou (1975). Idiotypic immunoglobulin on monoclonal lymphocytes of human multiple myeloma. Clinical Res. Vol. XXIII: 408A (abstract).

2. Bennett, M. and R. A. Steeves (1970). Immunocompetent cell function in mice infected with Friend Leukemia Virus. J. Nat. Cancer Inst. 44:1107.

3. Chirigos, M. A., K. Perk, W. Tumer, B. Burka, and M. Gomez (1968). Increased oncogenicity of Murine Sarcoma Virus (Moloney) by coinfection with Murine Leukemia Virus. Cancer Res. 28:1055.

4. Dent, P. B., R. D. A. Peterson, and R. A. Good (1965). A defect in cellular immunity during the incubation period of passage A Leukemia in C_3H mice. Proc. Soc. Exp. Biol. Med. 119:869.

5. Dent, P. B., M. D. Cooper, L. N. Payne, J. J. Solomon, B. R. Burmester, and R. A. Good (1968). Pathogenesis of avian lymphoid leukosis. II. Immunologic reactivity during lymphoma genesis. J. Nat. Cancer Inst. 41:391.

6. Dent, P. B. (1972). Immunodepression by Oncogenic Viruses. Prog. Med. Virol. 14:1.

7. Deodhar, S. D. and T. Chiang (1970). Immunosuppression with Friend Virus in allogenic murine tumor system. Fed. Proc. 29:560.

8. Fahey, J. L. and J. M. Humphrey (1962). Effect of transplantable plasma-cell tumor on antibody response in mice. Immunology. 5:110.

9. Friedman, H. and W. S. Ceglowski (1969). Murine virus leukaemogenesis—Relation between susceptibility and immunodepression. Nature 224:131.

10. Giacomoni, D., V. Yakulis, S. R. Wang, A. Cooke, S. Dray, and P. Heller (1974). In-vitro conversion of normal mouse lymphocytes by plasmacytoma RNA to express idiotypic specificity on their surfaces characteristic of the plasmacytoma Ig. Cellular Immunol. 11:389.

11. Heller, P., V. Yakulis, N. Bhoopalam, N. Costea, V. Cabana, and R. D. Nathan (1972). Surface immunoglobulins on circulating lymphocytes in mouse and human plasmacytoma. Trans. Assoc. Am. Physician LXXV: 192.

12. Jerne, N. K. and A. A. Nordin (1963). Plaque formation in agar by single antibody producing cells. Science 140:405.

13. Kuff, E. L., N. A. Wivel, and K. K. Lueders (1968). The extraction of intracisternal A particles from a mouse plasma-cell tumor. Cancer Res. 28:2137.

14. Katzmann, J., D. Giacomoni, V. Yakulis, and P. Heller (1975). Characterization of two plasmacytoma fractions and their RNA capable of changing lymphocyte SIg (cell conversion). Cellular Immunol. 18:98.

15. Lindstrom, F. D., W. R. Hardy, B. J. Eberle, and R. C. Williams, Jr. (1973). Multiple myeloma and benign monoclonal gammopathy: differentiation by immunofluorescence of lymphocytes. Ann. Int. Med. 78:837.

16. Mortensen, R. F., W. S. Ceglowski, and H. Friedman (1974). Leukemia virus-induced immunosuppression X. Depression of T cell-mediated cytotoxicity after infection of mice with FLV. J. Immunol. 112:2077.

17. Odaka, T., H. Ishii, K. Yamaura, and T. Yamamoto (1966). Inhibitory effect of FLV infection on the antibody formation to sheep erythrocytes in mice. J. Exp. Med. 36:277.

18. Old, L. J., D. A. Clarke, B. Benacerraf, and M. Goldsmith (1960). The reticuloendothelial system and the neoplastic process. Ann. N.Y. Acad. Sci. 88:264.

19. Schneider, M. and J. F. Dore (1969). Effect of infection of Friend Leukemia Virus on the immuno-reaction of mice sensitive and resistant to this virus. Rev. Fr. Clin. Biol. 14:1010.

20. Tanapatchaiyapong, P. and S. Zolla (1974). Humoral immunosuppressive substance in mice bearing plasmacytomas. Science 186:748.

21. Wedderburn, N. and M. H. Salaman (1968). The immunodepressive effect of Friend Virus II reduction of splenic hemolysin-producing cells in primary and secondary response. Immunol. London 15:439.

22. Yakulis, V., V. Cabana, D. Giacomoni, and P. Heller (1973). Surface immunoglobulins of circulating lymphocytes in mouse plasmacytoma. III. The effect of plasmacytoma RNA on the immune response. Immunol. Commun. 2:129.

23. Yakulis, V., N. Bhoopalam, S. Shade, and P. Heller (1972). Surface immunoglobulins of circulating lymphocytes in mouse plasmacytoma. I. Characteristics of lymphocyte surface immunoglobulins. Blood 39:453.

24. Zisblatt, M. and F. Lilly (1972). The effect of immunosuppression on oncogenesis by MSV. Proc. Soc. Exp. Biol. Med. 141:1036.

CHAPTER 11

Characterization of Virion and Cell Surface Reactivities of Natural Immune Sera to Murine Leukemia Viruses

J. N. Ihle, J. C. Lee,
J. Longstreth, and M. G. Hanna, Jr.

I. INTRODUCTION

Murine leukemia virus-associated cell surface antigens have been classified by humoral cytotoxicity (20), indirect immunofluorescence, and more recently by immunoelectron microscopy (1, 2). These experiments defined two major categories of leukemia cell antigens, the G and FMR antigens. Mouse antisera specific for the FMR subgroup are cytotoxic against FMR group leukemia cells and show viral neutralizing activity. Absorption of these sera with intact virions removes neutralization activity but not cytotoxicity activity (22), whereas absorption with disrupted virions removes both activities (4). Cytotoxicity may be related to antibodies specific for the internal virion protein, p15 (25), which is unique to FMR viruses. The FMR antisera neutralization activity may be due to antibodies against the major virion glycoprotein (gp71).

Research supported by the National Cancer Institute under Contract NOI-CO-25423 with Litton Bionetics, Inc.

Gross leukemia virus antigens have also been examined, and a vast number of virion and cell surface reactivities have been defined by inhibition techniques using indirect immunofluorescent assays and immunoelectron microscopy (2). The relationship of these serologically defined reactivities to specific virion proteins is not known; however, the complexity of immunologic reactivity of heterologous antisera to purified virion proteins (i.e., type, group, and interspecies reactivities) suggests that GSA (Gross soluble antigen), GCSA (Gross cell surface antigen), and VEA (virus envelope antigen) reactivities may reside in only a few specific virion proteins.

One consequence of spontaneous expression of endogenous murine leukemia virus is the natural development of a chronic immune response (12). Using the same techniques, specificity of autogenous immune sera was studied in several strains of mice (19). Additional studies indicate that most natural sera react predominantly with the virion envelope proteins gp71, gp43, and p15[E] (virion envelope) (10). The virion protein gp71 has been purified from Friend and Rauscher leukemia viruses (18, 24) and its serologic properties examined by heterologous antisera. These studies demonstrate that antisera to gp71 have complement-independent neutralizing activity (13, 23) as well as group-specific and type-specific reactivity. Similarly, serologic reactivity of these antisera with various viruses shows type-specific and group-specific as well as interspecies reactivity (9). Group- and type-specific reactivity also occurs with unfixed leukemia cells using immunofluorescent techniques (13), suggesting that this component is located on the cell surface.

The p15 protein reacting with natural immune sera corresponds to the p15[E] virion protein purified from Friend leukemia virus (11). Heterologous antisera to this virion protein show strong interspecies reactivity (21). This component is apparently completely different from p15, a protein of similar molecular weight purified from Rauscher leukemia virus (25). This protein induces heterologous antisera that react specifically with Rauscher and Friend virus and to a lesser extent with Moloney virus, but only weakly with other murine leukemia viruses. This suggests that this protein partially specifies the FMR subgroup.

II. EXPERIMENTAL DATA

The viruses used in the study reported here include: AKR virus isolated from an established line of AKR mouse embryo cells (FIC2(16a)) (obtained initially from Dr. W. P. Rowe, National Institutes of Health) that had spontaneously initiated virus synthesis; Moloney leukemia virus isolated from a chronically infected continuous-passage Swiss mouse embryo cell line (SME); Rauscher MuLV purified from the JLS-V5 cell line; RD-114 virus isolated from the RD cell line; rat leukemia virus isolated from a W/Fu rat cell line productively infected with rat leukemia virus; and Friend virus, obtained from Dr. D. B. Bolognesi, Duke University, Durham, N. C.

The radioimmune precipitation assay against intact radioactively labeled AKR virus has been described in detail (12). To prepare immune precipitates for SDS-polyacrylamide gel electrophoresis, 25–50 μl of serum were reacted with 2×10^5 cpm of Triton-disrupted virus and subsequently precipitated with anti-γ-globulin (10).

SDS-polyacrylamide gel electrophoresis was performed as

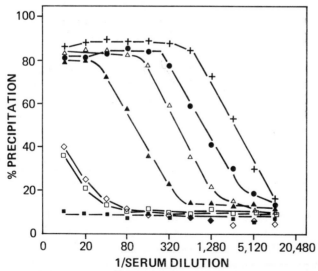

Figure 1. Radioimmune precipitation assay of various immune sera from 1-yr-old mice against [³H]leucine-labeled AKR leukemia virus. RF (▲——▲), B6C3F₁ (+——+), AKR (□——□), normal rabbit serum (■——■), C57BL/6 (●——●), NIH (◇——◇), and BALB/c (△——△).

described by Weber and Osborn (26). An indirect immunoferritin labeling technique was used for immunoelectron microscopy. The existence of natural antibodies to murine leukemia viruses was first clearly demonstrated by a quantitative and sensitive radio-immune precipitation assay (12). The curves obtained when age-matched sera from mice of various strains were titered against [³H]leucine-labeled AKR Gross type virus are shown in Figure 1. There was considerable diversity in the level of natural antibodies specific for endogenous leukemia virus. High titers of antibody were found in strains with low natural incidences of leukemia. Strains with low titers (AKR, RF) had either a high spontaneous incidence of leukemia or were those that have not yet been demon-strated to have the endogenous ecotropic virus (NIH, SWR/J). Titer variation appeared to correspond to immune responsiveness to the virus except in such strains as AKR and RF in which persistent viremia precludes a determination of total antibody levels. In all of our subsequent experiments, sera from B6C3F₁ animals (C57BL/6 ♀ × C3H/Anf ♂) were used to examine antigenic specificity of natural sera. These animals have a low natural incidence of lymphoma (< 5%) and are resistant to Gross virus-induced neoplasia.

The results of studies to determine the virion proteins recog-nized by autogenous immune sera using normal 1.5-yr B6C3F₁ serum and [³H]leucine-labeled AKR virus are shown in Figure 2. Normal sera reacted with and precipitated virion proteins having molecular weights of approximately 68,000, 43,000, and 17,000 on SDS-polyacrylamide gel electrophoresis. The 68,000 and the 17,000 molecular weight components correspond to gp71 and p15, respec-tively, by glucosamine labeling and competition assays using mono-specific antisera.

The ability of natural immune sera to cross react with other C-type viruses is shown in Figure 3. Various [³H]leucine-labeled viruses having similar radiospecific activities were prepared and used in radioimmunoassays with normal B6C3F₁ sera. This autogenous immune serum has comparable titers against various murine leukemia viruses (MuLV) including Moloney, Rauscher, and AKR viruses, but has no demonstrable titer against C-type viruses of other species including the endogenous cat leukemia virus (RD-114) and the rat leukemia virus (W/Fu). Natural sera react with both the G and FMR subgroups of MuLV and appear to have group-specific reactivity.

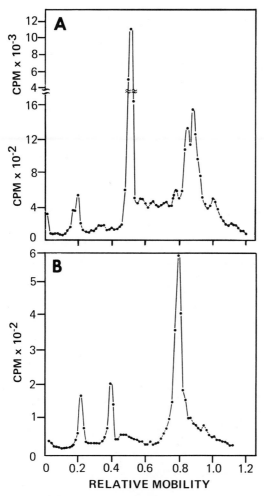

Figure 2. SDS-polyacrylamide gel electrophoresis profiles of (*A*) triton-disrupted [³H]leucine-labeled AKR MuLV; (*B*) immune precipitate of 1.5-year B6C3F₁ serum with triton-disrupted labeled AKR virus.

Figure 4*A* shows the SDS-polyacrylamide gel electrophoresis profile of immune precipitates of disrupted [³H]leucine-labeled Rauscher virus and normal B6C3F₁ serum. Similar to the AKR virus results, three peaks were observed with molecular weights of 68,000, 43,000, and 17,000, which appear to correspond to gp71, gp43, and p15. Figure 4*B* shows the results obtained with Moloney leukemia virus under identical conditions. Three peaks were

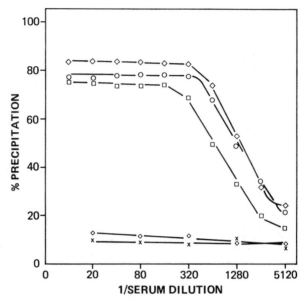

Figure 3. Radioimmune precipitation assay of 1.5-year B6C3F₁ sera against different intact [³H]leucine-labeled MuLV. Titration curves of natural immune serum to AKR MuLV (□ —— □), Rauscher MuLV (◇ —— ◇), Moloney MuLV (○ —— ○), rat leukemia virus (◇ —— ◇), and RD-114 (X —— X).

observed, corresponding to gp71, gp43, and p15. Thus, autogenous immune sera react with comparable virion proteins in both the G and FMR subgroups of MuLV.

Although the above results suggest that autogenous immune sera may recognize both G and FMR virion antigens equivalently, they do not rule out the possibility of weak cross reactions.

Figure 5 shows the results of a competition experiment in which unlabeled AKR virus was used to compete for the precipitation of [³H]leucine-labeled Rauscher, Moloney, and AKR virus. Unlabeled AKR virus was found to compete for the precipitation of radioactive AKR virus at limited dilutions of natural sera; 50% competition occurred with approximately 10 μg of unlabeled AKR virus, corresponding to a ratio of 20:1 (unlabeled to labeled virus). Similarly, unlabeled AKR virus competes for precipitation of labeled Moloney leukemia virus by normal sera, although the curve is displaced toward higher concentrations of AKR virus. The displacement may be due to differences in the specific activity of the labeled virus preparations or in the number of antigenic sites per virion.

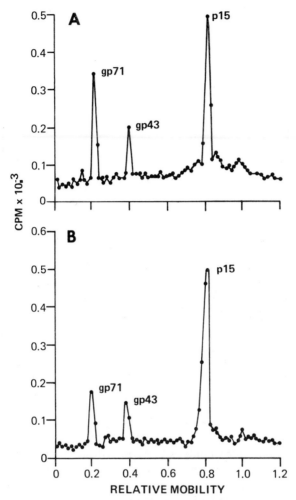

Figure 4. SDS-polyacrylamide gel electrophoresis profiles of (*A*) an immune precipitate of 1.5-year B6C3F$_1$ serum with Triton-disrupted [^{3}H]leucine-labeled Rauscher MuLV or (*B*) [^{3}H]leucine-labeled Moloney MuLV.

Similarity in slopes suggests comparable immune binding reactions. In contrast, AKR virus competes for precipitation of labeled Rauscher leukemia virus, indicating that natural immune sera only weakly cross react with this virus.

A second type of competition assay is shown in Figure 6. Neither Friend nor Rauscher virus at high concentrations was able

204   Ihle et al.

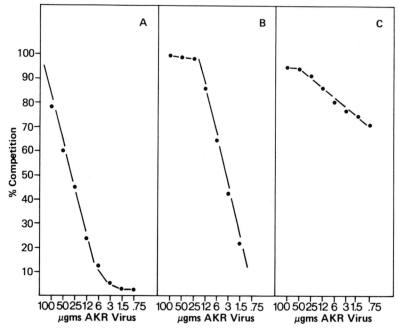

Figure 5. Inhibition of precipitation of labeled Moloney virus (*A*), labeled AKR virus (*B*), and labeled Rauscher virus (*C*), with B6C3F₁ serum by unlabeled AKR virus. B6C3F₁ serum diluted 1:128 was incubated for 1 hr at 37°C with various concentrations of unlabeled AKR virus. Labeled virus was then added and assayed as in the radioimmune precipitation assay.

to compete for precipitation of the labeled AKR virus. The AKR virus, however, was found to compete completely in the homologous reaction. Thus, the ability of AKR virus to compete for the precipitation of Rauscher leukemia virus and the inability of Rauscher or Friend virus to compete for precipitation of AKR virus, suggest that natural immune sera have specificity for Gross leukemia virus and do not cross react with Rauscher virus of the FMR group.

The efficacy of an autogenous immune response, particularly with regard to humoral cytotoxicity, may be dependent upon antigenic specificity for virion and cell surface proteins. Figure 7 shows the results obtained when rabbit antisera to gp71 and p15 were examined on K-36 cells by immunoelectron microscopy. Antisera to gp71 consistently reacted with budding virions as well as with portions of the cell membrane, whereas antisera to p15 reacted only with budding virions. Other cell lines were also examined. The results

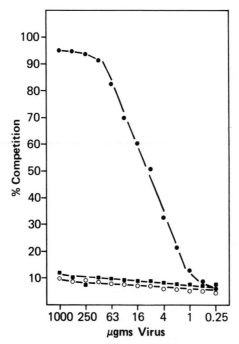

Figure 6. Inhibition of precipitation of labeled AKR virus by unlabeled AKR (● —— ●), Rauscher (○ —— ○), or Friend (■ —— ■) virus. B6C3F₁ serum was diluted 1:128, incubated 1 hr at 37°C with various concentrations of unlabeled AKR virus and then 1 μg (10,000 cpm) of labeled AKR virus was added. Samples were then treated as in the radioimmune precipitation assay.

are summarized in Table 1. Antisera to gp71 reacted with both the virion and cell membrane, whereas antisera to p15 reacted only with the budding virion in all the leukemia cell lines studied. Antisera to p30 reacted with the cell surface of EG2 cells but not with other leukemic cells. The location of p30 on the surface of some tumor cells has been previously suggested by immunofluorescence and cytotoxicity assays (6).

The reaction of normal B6C3F₁ serum with leukemic cells by immunoelectron microscopy is shown in Figure 8. Specific antibody was associated with the entire envelope of most budding and free C-type viruses. Unlike heterologous antisera to gp71, sera rarely show labeling on the leukemia cell surface. A possible explanation for this discrepancy is that the natural antigenic determinants recognized by B6C3F₁ serum are not exposed on the cell surface, whereas

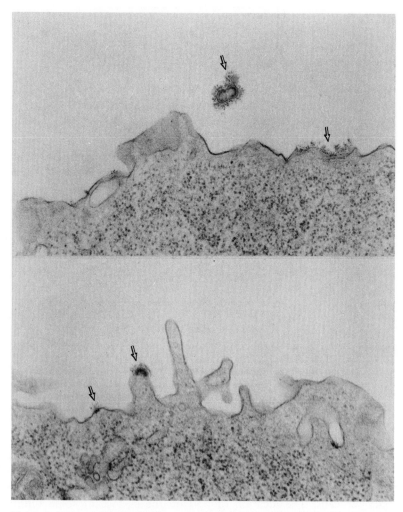

Figure 7. Immunoferritin labeling of AKR ascites leukemia K-36 cells. *Top,* cells were reacted with rabbit anti-gp71 then labeled with ferritin-conjugated goat anti-rabbit γ-globulin. Both cell surface and viral envelope are labeled. Bottom, cells reacted with rabbit anti-p15, then labeled with ferritin-conjugated goat anti-rabbit γ-globulin. Only the viral envelope is labeled. Both × 57,600.

the broader reactivity of the heterologous antisera recognizes the exposed determinants. Data supporting this hypothesis are summarized in Table 2. When heterologous antisera to gp71 are titrated by immunoelectron microscopy for cell surface versus virion

Table 1. Activity of rabbit immune sera towards murine leukemia cell lines[a]

Serum	EδG2		K-36		EL-4		FLC-745	
	VISA	VEA	VISA	VEA	VISA	VEA	VISA	VEA
Anti-gp71	+++	+++	+++	+++	+++	+++	+++	+++
Anti-p30	−	+++	−	−	−	−	−	−
Anti-p15	++++	−	−	+++	−	+++	−	+++

[a]Immunoferritin labeling of leukemia cell lines. +++ indicates an average of 6–8 ferritin positive sites per cell perimeter scored on more than 75% positive virions. A negative value is less than 2 ferritin labeled sites per cell perimeter or less than 10% positive virions.

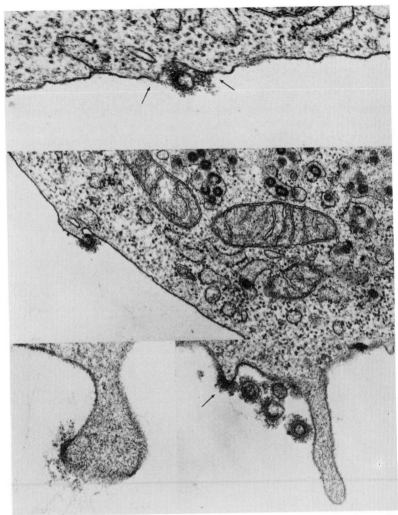

Figure 8. (A) Top, immunoferritin labeling of AKR mouse embryo cells spontaneously activated to produce RNA tumor virus. Cells were reacted with serum from normal B6C3F₁ mice and labeled with ferritin-conjugated rabbit anti-mouse γ-globulin. Entire envelope of free C-type particles is labeled. A small cellular projection (arrow), labeled, may be a budding virus whose nucleoid structure has not been resolved in this plane of section, or may be virus-mediated, nonvirion cell surface antigen. × 44,250. (B) Middle, gross virus-producing E ♂ G2 leukemia cells were reacted with immunoglobulin

Table 2. Titration of anti-gp71[a]

Antiserum dilution	Percent positive cells	Labeled sites/cell	Percent positive virus
1:4	80	6.0 ± 0.5	92
1:8	84	6.0 ± 0.6	88
1:16	60	4.1 ± 0.4	85
1:32	36	2.9 ± 0.4	89

[a]Immunoferritin labeling of K-36 cells using rabbit anti-gp71 at the dilutions indicated.

reactivity, the reaction with the cell surface is quickly lost, while at the same time the virion labeling remains constant. This suggests that the predominant immunologic reaction is with gp71 and that fewer antibodies exist that are capable of reacting with the antigenic determinants on the cell surface.

III. DISCUSSION

The results described above demonstrate that with a sensitive and quantitative radioimmune precipitation assay, an autogenous immune response can be demonstrated in a wide variety of mice (12, 19). The functionality of this immune response has been suggested by an inverse correlation between the incidence of spontaneous leukemia and antibody titers in various strains of mice known to harbor the ecotropic virus. Strains of mice having only the xenotropic virus and low natural antibody levels can be induced to produce higher levels of antibody by immunization with formalin-inactivated virus.

The efficacy of an immune response to the virus has been suggested by other observations. Hanna et al. (8) have demonstrated an inverse correlation between the degree of glomerulonephritis

eluted from kidneys of 2-year-old B6C3F$_1$ mice. Immunoferritin labeling of entire envelope of budding virus is demonstrated. × 1,000,000. (C) Bottom, immunoferritin labeling of C-type virus-producing BALB/c plasma cell tumor cells. Cells were reacted with serum from normal 14-week-old B6C3F$_1$ mice and labeled with ferritin-conjugated rabbit anti-mouse γ-globulin. Left, labeling of entire envelope of budding virus. Note large numbers of intracisternal particles characteristic of this cell line. × 55,000. Right, labeling of entire envelope of free virus that apparently has just completed budding from the cell. Limited regions of cell surface adjacent to budding site also are labeled (arrows). × 48,970.

(caused in part by immune complexes of C-type viruses) and the incidence of spontaneous leukemia in certain strains of mice. Similarly, Clapp and Yuhas (3) have shown an inverse correlation between glomerulonephritis and leukemia induction in irradiated RF mice. The variation in titers observed in several strains of mice appears to be due to immune responsiveness to the virus, which may be a function of the Rgv-1 gene previously described by Lilly (17). In particular, the Rgv-1 gene has been shown to confer resistance to Gross virus infection. This gene is localized on chromosome 17 in the H-2 region near the Ir locus. Compatible with an immune response, the Rgv-1 gene does not appear to influence virus expression. Its effect has not been seen in tissue culture and can be detected only at intermediate levels of virus expression.

An immune response may, however, depend upon qualitative as well as quantitative factors. As demonstrated here and by others (10), normal B6C3F$_1$ immune sera react primarily with the virion envelope proteins gp71, gp43, and p15. The predominant reaction is with gp71 followed by p15 and, last, with gp43 (11). The reaction with gp71 is significant because heterologous antisera to gp71 from Rauscher or Friend virus generally neutralize virus infectivity. In contrast, however, normal B6C3F$_1$ sera only weakly neutralize various murine ecotropic viruses but very effectively neutralize the xenotropic virus (7, 16).

The results demonstrate that natural immune sera from B6C3F$_1$ mice can cross react and precipitate leukemia viruses of both the G and FMR subgroups. The similarity in the titration curves for B6C3F$_1$ serum that is reacted with Moloney, Rauscher, or AKR virus, both in terms of titer and slopes, suggests a high degree of cross-reactivity. The ability of this serum to recognize comparable virion proteins in each of these viruses suggests that they are reacting equivalently.

Our competition experiments, however, clearly detected a lack of complete cross-reactivity. AKR virus competes more efficiently for the precipitation of Rauscher virus than in the homologous reaction. Similarly, Rauscher at high concentrations does not compete for AKR precipitation, suggesting that natural antibodies only weakly cross react with Rauscher virus. The Moloney virus has distinct antigenic differences from the Rauscher virus and appears to be comparable to the AKR virus. Thus, natural immune sera have group and type specificity but not interspecies reactivity.

The observation that natural antibodies to the endogenous virion gp71 do not react with cell surface antigens is highly significant. Immunoelectron microscopy with heterologous antisera provides evidence for the localization of gp71 on the cell surface and supports earlier findings by immunofluorescence (*13*) and antigen solubilization (*14*). Titration of heterologous sera against gp71 shows significant differences in titer for virion and cell surface labeling. This suggests that gp71 antigenic determinants exposed on the cell surface are not the same as those on the budding virion. It is suggested that the interspecies type determinants are expressed on the cell surface, but group-specific ones are not. Both types are thought to be expressed on budding and mature virions.

The absence of natural labeled antibodies on the cell surface may also be related to the above observations. Natural antibodies to gp71 have type-specific and weak group-specific activity as defined by our competition experiments. Furthermore, natural sera have low titers (1:10) against iodinated, purified gp71 from Friend or Rauscher virus, but high titers against purified gp71 from AKR virus. In terms of the biologic efficacy of this immune response, natural sera have not been demonstrated to have cytotoxicity against a variety of lymphoma cell lines (*7*). This suggests that reactivity with only budding virions is insufficient for detection of cytotoxicity. Therefore, natural sera are deficient in this sense because of limited reactivity with gp71. It will be interesting to determine whether or not immunizations with intact virus or virion specific proteins will alter the autogenous immune response so that additional biologic reactivities can be detected.

LITERATURE CITED

1. Aoki, T., R. B. Heberman, P. A. Johnson, M. Liu, and M. M. Sturm (1972). Wild-type gross leukemia virus: classification of soluble antigens (GSA). J. Virol. 10:1208–1219.
2. Aoki, T. and T. Takahashi (1972). Viral and cellular surface antigens of murine leukemias and myelomas. Serological analysis by immunoelectron microscopy. J. Exp. Med. 135:443–457.
3. Clapp, N. K. and J. M. Yuhas (1973). Suggested correlation between radiation-induced immunosuppression and radiogenic leukemia in mice. J. Nat. Cancer Inst. 51:1211–1215.
4. Friedman, M., F. Lilly, and S. G. Natheson (1974). Cell surface antigen induced by Friend murine leukemia virus is also in the virion. J. Virol. 14:1126–1131.

5. Gilden, R. V., S. Uroszlan, and R. Heubner (1971). Coexistence of intraspecies and interspecies specific antigenic determinants on the major structural polypeptide of mammalian C-type viruses. Nature New Biol. 231:107–108.

6. Grant, J. P., D. D. Bigner, P. J. Fischinger, and D. P. Bolognesi (1974). Expression of murine leukemia virus structural antigens on the surface of chemically-induced murine sarcomas. Proc. Nat. Acad. Sci. U.S.A. 71:5037–5041.

7. Hanna, M. G., Jr., J. N. Ihle, B. L. Batzing, R. W. Tennant, and C. K. Schenley (1975). Assessment of reactivities of natural antibodies to endogenous RNA tumor virus envelope antigens and virus-induced cell surface antigens. Cancer Res. 35:164–171.

8. Hanna, M. G., Jr., R. W. Tennant, J. M. Yuhas, N. K. Clapp, B. Batzing, and M. Snodgrass (1972). Autogenous immunity to endogenous RNA tumor virus in mice with a low natural incidence of lymphoma. Cancer Res. 32:2226–2234.

9. Hunsmann, G., V. Moennig, L. Pister, E. Seitert, and W. Schafer (1974). Properties of mouse leukemia viruses. VIII. The major viral glycoprotein of Friend leukemia virus: seroimmunological, interfering and hemagglutinating capacities. Virology 62:307–218.

10. Ihle, J. N., M. G. Hanna, L. E. Roberson, and F. T. Kenney (1974). Autogenous immunity to endogenous RNA tumor virus: identification of antibody reactivity to select viral antigens. J. Exp. Med. 136:1568–1581.

11. Ihle, J. N., M. G. Hanna, Jr., W. Schäfer, G. Hunsmann, D. P. Bolognesi, and G. Hüper (1975). Polypeptides of mammalian oncornaviruses. III. Localization of p15 and reactivity with natural antibody. Virology 63:60–67.

12. Ihle, J. N., M. Yurconic, Jr., and M. G. Hanna, Jr. (1973). Autogenous immunity to endogenous RNA tumor virus: radioimmune precipitation assay of mouse serum antibody levels. J. Exp. Med. 138:194–208.

13. Ikeda, H. T., T. Pineus, T. Yoshiki, M. Strand, J. T. August, E. A. Boyse, and R. C. Mellors (1974). Biological expression of antigenic determinants of murine leukemia virus proteins gp69/71 and p30. J. Virol. 14:1274–1280.

14. Kennel, S. J., B. C. Del Villano, R. L. Levy, and R. A. Lerner (1973). Properties of an oncornavirus glycoprotein: evidence for its presence on the surface of virions and infected cells. Virology 55:464–475.

15. Klein, E., and G. Klein (1964). Antigenic properties of lymphomas induced by the Moloney agent. J. Nat. Cancer Inst. 32:547–568.

16. Lee, J. C., M. G. Hanna, Jr., J. N. Ihle, and S. A. Aaronson (1974). Autogenous immunity to endogenous RNA tumor virus: differential reactivities of immunoglobulins M and G to virus envelope antigens. J. Virol. 14:773–781.

17. Lilly, F. 1966. The histocompatibility-2 locus and susceptibility to tumor induction. Nat. Cancer Inst. Monograph 22:631–641.

18. Moennig, V., H. Frank, G. Hunsmann, I. Schneider, and W. Schafer (1974). Properties of mouse leukemia viruses. VII. The major viral glycoprotein of Friend leukemia virus. Isolation and physio-chemical properties. Virology 61:100–111.

19. Nowinski, R. C. and S. L. Kaehler (1974). Antibody to leukemia virus: widespread occurrence in inbred mice. Science 185:869–871.

20. Old, L. J., E. A. Boyse, and E. Stockert (1964). Typing of mouse leukemias by serological methods. Nature 201:777–779.

21. Schäfer, W., G. Hunsmann, V. Moennig, F. DeNoronha, D. D. Bolognesi, R. W. Green, and G. Hüper (1975). Polypeptides of mammalian oncornaviruses. II. Characterization of a murine leukemia virus polypeptide (p15) bearing interspecies reactivity. Virology 63:48–59.

22. Steeves, R. A. 1968. Cellular antigen of Friend virus-induced leukemias. Cancer Res. 28:338–342.

23. Steeves, R. A., M. Strand, and J. T. August (1974). Structural proteins of mammalian oncogenic RNA viruses: murine leukemia envelope glycoprotein. J. Virol. 14:187–189.

24. Strand, M. and J. T. August (1973). Structural proteins of oncogenic ribonucleic acid viruses. II. A new interspecies antigen. J. Biol. Chem. 248:5627–5633.

25. Strand, M., R. Wilsnack, and J. T. August (1974). Structural proteins of mammalian oncogenic RNA viruses: immunological characterization of p15 polypeptide of Rauscher murine virus. J. Virol. 14:1575–1583.

26. Weber, K. and M. Osborn (1969). The reliability of molecular weight determinations by dodecyl-sulfate polyacrylamide gel electrophoresis. J. Biol. Chem. 244:4406–4412.

CHAPTER 12

Restoration of Immunocompetence in Leukemia Virus-Infected Splenocytes in vitro by Peritoneal Exudate Macrophages

S. Specter, M. Bendinelli,
N. Patel, and H. Friedman

I. INTRODUCTION

Murine leukemia viruses (MuLV) are able to alter the immuno-competence of mouse splenocytes both in vivo (5–7) and in vitro (9, 11, 12). However, the mechanism by which this alteration occurs is poorly understood. The studies reported below were designed to determine whether a particular cell population from uninfected mice can restore immunocompetence to MuLV-infected splenocytes cultured in Marbrook chambers in vitro (10).

Two viruses were used in this study: (a) Rowson-Parr virus (RPV), a lymphatic leukemia virus (LLV), isolated by endpoint dilution of Friend leukemia virus (FLV); and (b) the FLV complex containing both the LLV and spleen focus forming virus (SFFV) components. Both viruses were demonstrated to be free of lactic dehydrogenase virus and lymphocytic choriomeningitis virus (1, 3).

II. EXPERIMENTAL DESIGN

Virus was injected intravenously into BALB/c mice and their spleens were removed at various time intervals after infection. Single-cell

216		Specter et al.

suspensions were made, and 5×10^6 cells were cultured with 2×10^6 sheep erythrocytes (SRBC) in Marbrook chambers for 5 days at 37°C in 5% CO_2. Cells were removed and plated by the technique of Jerne et al. (8). At the time of culture initiation in experimental groups, graded numbers of normal cells from one of several sources were added to the infected splenocytes.

III. EXPERIMENTAL DATA

Table 1 shows that peak immunosuppression of RPV-infected spleen cells occurred at 5 days postinfection; with FLV the immunosuppression was progressive, increasing with longer time of infection. Both viruses produced splenocytes that were capable of greatly reducing the PFC response to SRBC; 10^5 infected cells suppressed 5×10^6 normal splenocytes when cocultivated in vitro.

As seen in Table 2, when peritoneal exudate cells (PEC) are added to 5-day post-RPV-infected splenocytes, 10^5–10^6 cells restore immunocompetence, with the peak response occurring with 3×10^5 cells. The exudates contain 80–85% macrophages. When exudate cells are treated with anti-θ serum and complement to remove T cells, activity is not altered, indicating that the cells responsible for restoration are macrophages (Figure 1). However, when adherent

Table 1. Primary immune response in vitro of uninfected splenocytes in the presence of Rowson-Parr and Friend leukemia virus-infected splenocytes

Infected donor mice[a]	PFC response[b]	PFC response of normal cells[c]	
		− Infected cells	+ Infected cells
RPV			
5 days	148[d]	2,225	1,184
15 days	1,477	2,225	713
36 days	1,123	2,225	561
FLV (29 days)	132	700	283

[a]Spleen cell donors infected with either RPV or FLV on day indicated before day of in vitro culture initiation.

[b]Direct PFC response of 5×10^6 spleen cells from indicated mouse group immunized in vitro with RBC for 5 days.

[c]Direct PFC response of 5×10^6 normal spleen cells immunized in vitro with RBC for 5 days in the presence or absence of 10^5 of the indicated infected spleen cells.

[d]PFC per 10^6 viable cells recovered from 3–5 cultures.

Table 2. PFC response in vitro of Rowson-Parr virus-infected splenocytes after addition of uninfected peritoneal exudate and adherent spleen cells

Additional uninfected cells		Number of added cells per culture[a]					
Source	PFC[b]	0	3×10^3	3×10^4	1×10^5	3×10^5	1×10^6
Peritoneal exudate cells	0	135	149	324	724	1020	N.D.
Adherent spleen cells	65	88	94	162	N.D.	236	312

[a]Average number of plaque forming cells per 10^6 viable cells recovered for 5–6 spleen cell cultures from 5-day RPV-infected mice with indicated cells and SRBC for 5 days.

[b]5×10^6 cells cultured alone with SRBC only for 5 days in vitro.

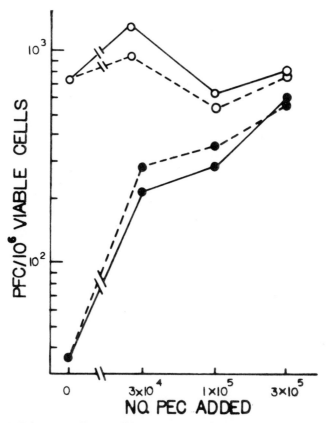

Figure 1. Primary antibody PFC response in vitro of uninfected and 5-day Rowson-Parr virus-infected splenocytes in the presence of uninfected peritoneal exudate cells pretreated with AKR normal (*broken line*) or anti-θ (*continuous line*) serum. Each point represents the average PFC response of 3–5 cultures tested in duplicate.

cells (a macrophage-rich population) are added to infected splenocytes they are totally incapable of restoring immunocompetence. This may be due to the need for an activated macrophage to enable the infected splenocytes to respond. The PEC represents an activated population whereas the spleen macrophages may not be activated.

Similar results are obtained to those with the RPV infected cells using FLV infected splenocytes (Table 3). 3×10^5 PEC causes the optimal restoration of responsiveness to SRBC in vitro; partial restoration is achieved when 10^5–10^6 PEC are added to the FLV-infected spleen cell cultures.

Table 3. PFC response in vitro of Friend leukemia virus-infected splenocytes after addition of uninfected peritoneal exudate cells

Spleen cells added	Number of added P.E. cells per culture[a]					
	0^b	3×10^3	3×10^4	1×10^5	3×10^5	1×10^6
FLV (20 days)	82	123	168	361	386	279
Normal (control)	592	—	—	—	—	—

[a] Average number of PFC per 10^6 viable cells recovered for 6–8 spleen cell cultures.
[b] 5×10^6 cells cultured with SRBC for 5 days.

The ability to restore immunocompetence to RPV-infected splenocytes rests solely with the PEC population, as recorded in Table 4. Populations of bone marrow (B) derived cells, thymus (T) derived cells, whole spleen cells from normal mice, and SRBC "educated" T cells all are incapable of restoring immunity to the RPV-suppressed spleen cells. The failure of these cell populations to enhance responsiveness is further evidence that the responsible cells in the PEC are macrophages.

IV. DISCUSSION

The mechanism by which macrophages can restore responsiveness is not certain. We believe that improved antigen "focusing" or "processing" is occurring. Four observations support this hypothesis:

Table 4. Effect of addition of unifected lymphoid cells from various sources on the primary PFC response in vitro of Rowson-Parr virus-infected splenocytes

Additional uninfected cells		Numbers of added normal cells per culture			
Source	PFC[a]	0	1×10^3	1×10^5	2×10^6
Thymus	0	76^b	0.141	141	182
Bone marrow	40		79	123	228
Spleen	950		172	135	276
RBC educated T cells	104	211	73	65	147

[a] Response of 5×10^6 cells cultured alone with SRBC for 5 days in vitro.
[b] Average number of plaque forming cells per 10^6 viable cells recovered for 3–5 cultures 5 days after immunization with SRBC.

1. Increasing antigen concentration enables RPV-infected cells to respond to the antigen without the addition of helper PEC (2).

2. *Escherichia coli* lipopolysaccharide, which stimulates macrophage phagocytic activity, as well as other functions of immunologically active cells, enhances the SRBC response of infected cells to the level of normal splenocytes (2).

3. 2-Mercaptoethanol (2-ME), which replaces the macrophages ability to enhance lymphocyte viability, is not effective in restoring immunocompetence, indicating that the macrophage has an active role in this response.

4. 10^7 PEC injected into FLV-infected mice was not capable of restoring immunocompetence to these mice, when they were tested for humoral response to SRBC (4). The PEC probably need to be in intimate contact with the infected splenocytes to focus antigen for their response, thus explaining the in vivo failure. Experiments are in progress to determine whether or not the immunologic dysfunction in infected animals is occurring at the level of the macrophage.

LITERATURE CITED

1. Bendinelli, M. (1973). Immunodepression by Rowson-Parr Virus. *In:* Virus Tumorigenesis and Immunogenesis, W. S. Ceglowski and H. Friedman, Eds., p. 181. Academic Press, New York.
2. Bendinelli, M., G. Kaplan, and H. Friedman (1975). Reversal of Leukemia Virus-Induced Immunosuppression In Vitro: The Role of Peritoneal Macrophages. Submitted for publication.
3. Ceglowski, W. S. and H. Friedman (1968). Immunosuppression by Leukemia Viruses. I. Effect of Friend Disease Virus on Cellular and Humoral Hemolysin Responses of Mice to a Primary Immunization with Sheep Erythrocytes. J. Immunol. 101:594–604.
4. Ceglowski, W. S. and H. Friedman (1975). Failure of Peritoneal Exudate Macrophages to Reverse Immunologic Impairment by Friend Leukemia Virus. Proc. Soc. Exp. Biol. Med. 148:808–812.
5. Dent, P. B. (1972). Immunodepression by Oncogenic Viruses. Prog. Med. Virol. 14:1–35.
6. Friedman, H. and W. S. Ceglowski (1974). Virus Tumorigenesis and Immunity: Influence of Immunostimulation and Immunodepression. *In:* Virus Tumorigenesis and Immunogenesis in The Role of Immunologic Factors in Viral and Oncogenic Processes. R. F. Beers, Jr., and R. C. Tilghman, Eds., p. 187–209. Johns Hopkins Univ. Press, Baltimore. Md.
7. Gross, L. (1970). Oncogenic Viruses, 2d ed. Pergammon Press, London.

8. Jerne, N. K., A. A. Nordin, and C. Henry (1963). The Agar Plaque Technique for Recognizing Antibody Producing Cells. *In:* Cell Bound Antibodies, B. Amos and H. Koprowski, Eds., p. 109. The Wistar Inst. Press, Philadelphia, Pa.

9. Kateley, J. R., I. Kamo, G. Kaplan, and H. Friedman (1974). Suppressive Effect of Leukemia Virus-Infected Lymphoid Cells on In Vitro Immunization of Normal Splenocytes. J. Nat. Cancer Inst. 53:1371–1378.

10. Marbrook, J. (1967). Primary Immune Response In Vitro of Spleen Cells. Lancet 2:1279.

11. Specter, S. and H. Friedman (1975). Immunosuppression In Vitro by Cell-Free Homogenates of Friend Virus Infected Spleens. Fed. Proc. 34:866.

12. Weislow, O. S. and E. F. Wheelock (1975). Depression of Humoral Immunity to Sheep Erythrocytes In Vitro by Friend Virus Leukemia Spleen Cells: Induction of Resistance by Statolon. J. Immunol. 114:211–215.

CHAPTER 13

Assignment of Gene(s) for Cell Transformation and Malignancy to Human Chromosome 7 Carrying the SV40 Genome

C. M. Croce

I. INTRODUCTION

There is a concordant segregation of the expression of SV40 T antigen and the presence of human chromosome 7 in somatic cell hybrids between mouse cells deficient in thymidine kinase and LN-SV SV40-transformed human cells (*1, 3–5*). SV40 can be rescued only from the clones that are SV40 T antigen-positive and contain human chromosome 7, but not from those that have lost this human chromosome (*1, 3, 4*). Subcloning of SV40 T antigen-positive hybrid clones results in the isolation of SV40 T antigen-positive and negative subclones; all the SV40 T antigen-positive subclones contain human chromosome 7, and all the SV40 T antigen-negative subclones are without this chromosome (*5*). Fusion

This work was supported in part by United States Public Health Service research Grants CA 10815 and CA 16685 from the National Cancer Institute, RR 05540 from the Division of Research Resources, GM 20700 from the Institute of General Medical Sciences, and by a Basil O'Connor Starter Grant to the author from the National Foundation. The author is a recipient of Research Career Development Award CA 00143 from the National Cancer Institute.

of the hybrid subclones with African green monkey cells results in the rescue of SV40 only from the subclones that contain human chromosome 7, and not from those that have lost this chromosome (3). Therefore, the SV40 genome is integrated in, or attached to, human chromosome 7 in the SV40-transformed cell line LN–SV.

The SV40 DNA present in the hybrid clones has been quantitated by two different methods of nucleic acid hybridization (10). Reassociation kinetics as well as hybridization with a single-strand probe show a positive correlation between the number of copies of SV40 DNA and the number of copies of human chromosome 7 present in the hybrid cells (10).

The results below were determined from studies designed to demonstrate whether or not the human chromosome 7 that carries the SV40 genomes contains gene(s) responsible for the expression of the transformed phenotype in vitro and the malignant phenotype in vivo. Therefore normal mouse cells (peritoneal macrophages) were hybridized with LN–SV SV40-transformed human cells. The resulting hybrid cells were examined for the expression of the transformed and malignant phenotypes and for the presence of human chromosomes.

II. EXPERIMENTAL DATA

Techniques used in these experiments have been previously described (6, 10, 12–14). From 1 to 4×10^7 cells per mouse were injected into nude mice of a BALB/c background. Tumors were removed at various times (3 weeks to 3 months after injection) and transferred to culture. Identification of the chromosomes present in the hybrid cells and in the tumor cells was established following Giemsa banding staining according to a modification of the method described by Seabright (2, 17). At least 20 metaphases for each hybrid clone or tumor cell line were photographed and analyzed.

All 168 clones between LN-SV cells and C57BL/6 (111 clones) and BALB/c (6) mouse peritoneal macrophages expressed SV40 T antigen (Table 1). Sixty-seven of these clones were studied for the presence of human chromosomes and for the expression of the transformed phenotype, as determined by colony formation in soft agar and methylcellulose. As shown in Figure 1, all the hybrid cell clones were transformed (> 1 colony per 100 cells seeded in soft agar and in methylcellulose). All the hybrid cells contained at

Table 1. Presence of SV40 T antigen in hybrid clones between mouse peritoneal macrophages and SV40-transformed human fibroblasts

Hybrid cells			No. of hybrid clones studied	No. of clones showing presence of SV40 T antigen[a]
Mouse	×	Human		
C57BL/6	×	LN–SV	111	111
Balb/c	×	LN–SV	57	57

[a]One hundred percent of cells of each clone were positive for SV40 T antigen.

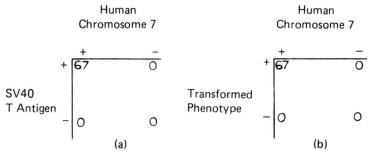

Figure 1. Positive correlation between the expression of the SV40 T antigen (a) and that of the transformed phenotype (b) and the presence of the human chromosome 7 in 67 independent hybrid clones between C57BL/6 and BALB/c MPM and LN-SV cells. Forty-five of the analyzed hybrid clones were between C57BL/6 MPM and LN-SV cells and 22 between BALB/c MPM and LN-SV cells. At least one human chromosome 7 was present in all the metaphases examined.

least one copy of human chromosome 7 (Figure 1). In 13 of the 67 hybrid cell clones analyzed, human chromosome 7 was the only human chromosome present in the hybrid cells.

A C57BL × LN-SV hybrid cell population containing 14 different human chromosomes (Table 2) was injected into 20 nude mice (9, 16, 18) (2–4 × 10⁷ cells per mouse). The tumors, which developed in 5 of these mice, were transferred to tissue culture and analyzed for the expression of SV40 T antigen and presence of human chromosomes. The results of these studies are shown in Table 3; the human chromosome 7 was retained by 100% of the tumor cells examined (Table 3 and Figure 2). Reinoculation of the tumor cell lines into nude mice resulted in the formation of tumors in all mice injected (17). Twenty-two nude mice were also

Table 2. Presence of different human chromosomes in hybrid cells between C57BL/6 peritoneal macrophages and LN = SV cells

Human chromosome	Frequency in hybrids (%)[a]	Human chromosome	Frequency in hybrids (%)[a]
4	5.9	13	5.9
5	60.8	14	7.8
6	70.6	15	17.6
7	100[b]	16	2.0
9	5.9	17	60.8
11	54.9	18	3.9
12	23.5	20	5.9

[a]A total of 51 metaphases examined.
[b]On the average the hybrid cells contained 2.3 chromosomes 7 per cell.

injected with near-diploid hybrid clones (53-87-3 Cl 10 and 53-87-3 CI 43), between BALB/c mouse peritoneal macrophages and LN-SV cells (10^7 cells per mouse) (Table 4) (8). Twenty mice developed large tumors (the remaining 2 mice died a few days after the injection). Six tumors were transferred to culture and analyzed for the expression of SV40 T antigen and the presence of human chromosomes. As shown in Table 4, all 6 tumor lines retained at least one copy of human chromosome 7. The karyologic analysis of the tumor lines also showed that a single copy of human chromosome 7 was present in 2 of the tumorigenic hybrid lines (8), indicating that the presence of a single copy of human chromosome 7 carrying the SV40 genome is sufficient for the expression of the malignant phenotype in the hybrid cells.

III. DISCUSSION

The fusion of normal nondividing mouse cells (mouse peritoneal macrophages) with LN-SV SV40-transformed human cells resulted in the formation of hybrid cells that retained the human chromosome 7 carrying the SV40 genome. Since no hybrid clones were found that did not contain at least a copy of human chromosome 7, we infer that this chromosome is necessary for the growth of the hybrid cells.

Sixty-seven independent hybrid clones were tested for colony formation in semisolid media. All of them were found to originate colonies when seeded in soft agar and in methylcellulose. These

Table 3. Karyologic analysis of cells recovered from tumors induced in "nude" mice by inoculation of hybrid cells

Source of tumors	No. of days after inoculation before removal	Cells showing SV40 T antigen (%)	Human chromosomes[a]						
			5	6	7	11	17		
"Nude" 1	22	100	8/45	35/45	45/45	0/45	0/45		
"Nude" 2	28	100	0/30	21/30	30/30	0/30	0/30		
"Nude" 4	42	100	0/39	25/39	39/39	1/39	15/39		
"Nude" 7	70	100	0/26	10/26	26/26	0/26	1/26		
"Nude" 8	76	100	0/33	3/33	33/33	0/33	0/33		

[a]Numbers of metaphases showing presence of this chromosome over total analyzed.

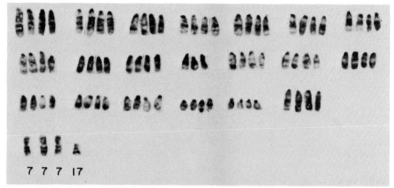

7 7 7 |7

Figure 2. Karyotype of a hybrid cell derived from "nude" 4 tumor. The hybrid cell contains a quasi-tetraploid number of mouse chromosomes and four human chromosomes (three chromosomes 7 and one chromosome 17).

experiments indicate that the transformed phenotype is dominant in somatic cell hybrids between normal mouse cells and SV40-transformed human cells and that the human chromosome 7 carrying the SV40 genome is responsible for the expression of the transformed phenotype in vitro. Different hybrids were then injected into nude mice, in which heterotransplantation of human tumors can be successfully achieved (9, 16, 18). Since the hybrid cell lines tested were found to be tumorigenic in nude mice, and since all the tumor cell lines derived from the tumors contained the human chromosome 7 carrying the SV40 genome, we conclude that the malignant phenotype is dominant in this type of hybrids and that the human chromosome 7 carrying the SV40 genome is also responsible for the expression of the malignant phenotype in vivo.

The hybridization of normal mouse cells with different human cancer cells might result in the formation of transformed and tumorigenic hybrid cells that selectively retain the human chromosome(s) responsible for malignancy. This could allow the identification of the human chromosome(s) involved in the control of the cancer phenotype and a better understanding of the genetics of cancer in man.

LITERATURE CITED

1. Croce, C. M., A. J. Girardi, and H. Koprowski (1973). Proc. Nat. Acad. Sci. U.S.A. 70:3617–3620.

Table 4. Correlation of the expression of SV40 T antigen and the presence of human chromosome 7 in tumorigenic hybrid clones and tumor cells

Cells	T antigen-positive cells (%)	Human chromosomes (av. no. per cell)			Rearranged chromosome 7 (av. no. per cell)	Mouse chromosomes (no. per cell)		No. metaphases analyzed[a]
		5	7	11		Average	Range	
1. 53-87 (3) clone 10	100	0	1.0	0	0	41.9	39–44	25
2. Nu10 IT (1)	100	0	1.3	0	0.6	41.8	38–44	49
3. Nu10 IT (2)	100	0	1.0	0	0.1	42.0	40–43	27
4. 53-87(3) clone 43	100	0.9	1.2	0.5	0	40.3	39–42	30
5. Nu43 IT (1)	100	0.6	1.1	0.3	0.1	41.1	39–43	39
6. Nu43 IT (2)	100	0.1	2.0	0	0	41.4	38–44	24
7. Nu43 IT (3)	100	0.1	1.9	0	0.1	41.6	40–43	37
8. Nu43 IT (4)	100	0.2	2.6	0	0.0	40.3	39–42	39
9. Nu43 IT (5)	100	0.4	1.9	0.2	0.1	41.8	39–47	55

[a]Less than 10% of the cells of 53-87 (3) clone 10, Nu10 IT. (1) and Nu10 IT. (2) were near tetraploid and they were not included in the computation of the averages. Less than 20% of the cells of 53-87 (3) clone 43 and its tumor derivatives were near tetraploid and they were not included in the computation of the averages.

2. Croce, C. M., B. B. Knowles, and H. Koprowski (1973). Exp. Cell Res. 82:457–461.
3. Croce, C. M., K. Huebner, A. J. Girardi, and H. Koprowski (1974). Virology 60:276–281.
4. Croce, C. M., K. Huebner, A. J. Girardi, and H. Koprowski (1974). Cold Spring Harbor Symp. Quant. Biol. 39:335–343.
5. Croce, C. M. and H. Koprowski (1974). J. Exp. Med. 139:1350–1353.
6. Croce, C. M. and H. Koprowski (1974). J. Exp. Med. 140:1221–1229.
7. Croce, C. M., D. Aden, and H. Koprowski (1975). Proc. Nat. Acad. Sci. U.S.A. 72:1397–1400.
8. Croce, C. M., D. Aden, and H. Koprowski (1975). Science 190:1200–1202.
9. Flanagan, S. P. (1966). Genet. Res. 8:295–309.
10. Khoury, G. and C. M. Croce (1975). Cell 6:535–542.
11. Klinger, H. P. (1972). Cytogenetics 11:424–435.
12. Littlefield, J. W. (1964). Science 145:709–710.
13. Macpherson, I. (1969). In: Fundamental Techniques in Virology, K. Habel and N. Salzman, Eds., pp. 214–219. Academic Press, New York.
14. Pope, J. H. and W. P. Rowe (1964). J. Exp. Med. 120:121–128.
15. Risser, R. and R. Pollack (1974). Virology 59:477–489.
16. Rygaard, J. and C. O. Povlsen (1969). Acta Pathol. Microbiol. Scand. 77:758–760.
17. Seabright, M. (1971). Lancet 2:971–972.
18. Visfeldt, J., C. O. Povlsen, and J. Rygaard (1972). Acta Pathol. Microbiol. Scand. 80A:169–176.

CHAPTER 14

Surface Morphology of Spleen Cells from Mice Infected with Friend Leukemia Virus

P. A. Farber,
S. Specter, and H. Friedman

I. INTRODUCTION

Infection of susceptible strains of mice with Friend leukemia virus
(FLV) results in a massive splenomegaly with proliferation of
abnormal cells in the spleen and other lymphoid organs (7, 16, 17).
The rapid neoplastic proliferation of primitive cells of the red pulp
of the spleen is associated with a marked and generalized immunosuppression (5). Previous electron microscope studies have shown
the presence of C-type particles in immature blast-like lymphoid
cells (3, 9, 10). These virus particles have also been observed
budding from the surface of plasma cells actively secreting antibodies
to sheep erythrocytes. Additional studies have indicated that the
B cell is the main target of FLV-induced immunosuppression (6,
8). There is a marked decrease in spleen cells bearing surface
immunoglobulins and a depression in the capping response of these
immunoglobulin-bearing cells during FLV infection.

Recently, the scanning electron microscope (SEM) has been
used to study cell surface architecture. Initially it was thought that
B and T lymphocytes could be differentiated on the basis of their
surface topography, since the B cells possess numerous surface
projections, or villi, and the T cells have a generally smooth surface
with a few digitations (11, 13–15). Such dichotomies in surface
appearance between B and T cells have not been confirmed by
other laboratories (1, 12). This controversy does not, however,

diminish the usefulness of the SEM in detecting subtle alterations of cellular morphology during the infectious process.

The present study was initiated to study the surface characteristics of murine splenocytes and possible changes that may occur during infection with Friend leukemia virus. These alterations might then be related to the infectious process and the development of immunosuppression.

II. EXPERIMENTAL DATA

BALB/c mice were inoculated intravenously with a stock preparation of Friend leukemia virus (FLV). At various times after infection

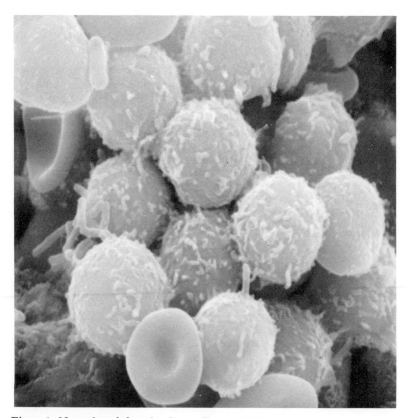

Figure 1. Normal, uninfected spleen cells.   x 6,500.

representative animals were sacrificed and single-cell suspensions obtained from their spleens. Splenic lymphocytes were further purified by Ficoll-Hypaque centrifugation. Cells were fixed for 1 hr in 1% glutaraldehyde and postfixed in 1% osmium tetroxide for 15 min, washed, and dried by the critical point method (2). The membranes were mounted on aluminum studs, coated with carbon and gold-paladium, and examined with an Etec autoscan microscope operating at 20 kv (Etec Corp., Hayward, Ca.).

Normal BALB/c splenocytes show the expected spectrum of cell types as previously described by Polliack (15). Most cells have numerous villous projections on their surface. A smaller percentage have smooth topography or only a few villi. The appearance of these cells is shown in Figure 1.

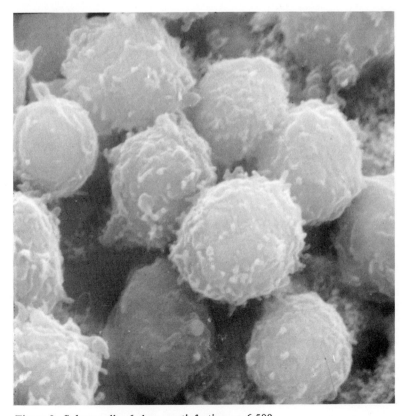

Figure 2. Spleen cells, 6 days postinfection. x 6,500.

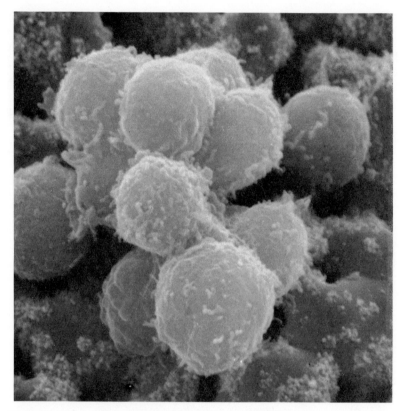

Figure 3. Spleen cells, 10 days postinfection. x 6,500.

Within a few days after infection with FLV a significant change occurs in the surface characteristics of the splenic lymphocytes. There is a decrease in the number of villous covered cells and an increase in the number of smooth cells. By 6 days the percentage of villous covered lymphocytes decreases to 29% while smooth cells increase to 31%. Cells with a few villi (intermediate) increase to 40% (Figure 2). The number of smooth lymphocytes increased as the FLV infection progressed. By 10 days most cells show a smooth configuration (Figure 3). By 17 days after infection few normal lymphocytes are present. All of the splenocytes from infected animals are smoother and larger than normal lymphocytes (Figure 4). Many of these cells possess blebs on their surfaces, reminiscent of the "knobs" described by deHarven et al. (4) in

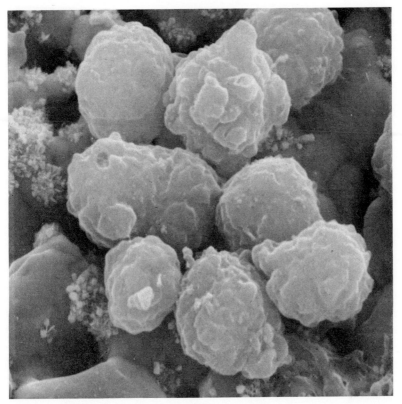

Figure 4. Spleen cells, 17 days postinfection. x 6,500.

their SEM study of cells continuously infected with FLV (Figure 5). Later in the infection (30 days postinoculation) there are lymphocytes with numerous blebs as well as punctate lesions resembling holes (Figure 6). These pores seem to coalesce so that at this late stage lysed lymphocytes are present.

III. DISCUSSION

Previous studies with the transmission electron microscope have shown the presence of lymphoblastoid cells with both intracellular and budding C-type virus particles in infected mice. These findings are confirmed and extended by using the scanning electron microscope. During the first days following FLV infection there is a

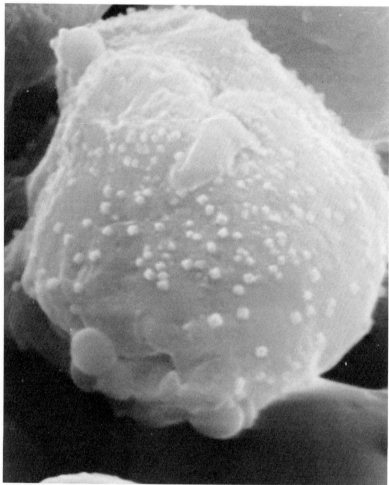

Figure 5. Splenic Lymphocyte, 35 days postinfection. x 22,000.

discernible change in the surface characteristics of splenic lymphocytes. Smoother, larger lymphocytes appear in the spleen; these
increase in number as the infection progresses. Concomitantly, there
is a decrease in villous-covered lymphocytes which some believe
to be the B-lymphocyte. These early changes occur before splenomegaly and the increase in spleen cell number. The immunosuppression that occurs during FLV infection has been extensively
investigated and is believed to affect mainly B cell function. If one

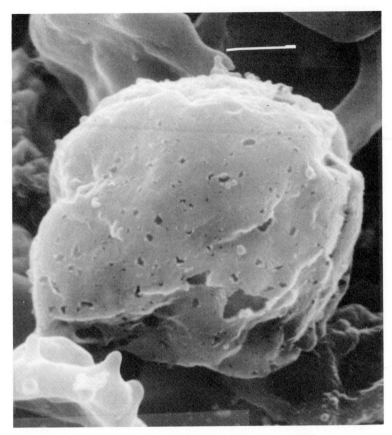

Figure 6. Splenic lymphocyte, 30 days after infection. x 7,000.

believes that villous-covered lymphocytes are indeed B lymphocytes, then the present findings that show a decrease in these cells early in FLV-infection are confirmatory of the loss of B function. The mechanism for this preferential block may be the infection and lysis of B cells or their precursors by virus. However, T cell function derangements have also been seen with FLV, which argues against any specificity of the virus for B cells. The appearance or large cells with smooth surfaces that increase in number and eventually form the predominant cell type is characteristic of FLV infection in the spleen. Surface blebs that appear to be budding virus are seen in many of these cells. Eventually, surface lesions appear that may represent injury to the cell by virus or may represent host-induced cell injury through the immune response. Complement-mediated cell lysis may result from the new viral antigens that occur on infected cells. Cytotoxic lymphocytes may also cause such lesions.

There is some controversy on the significance of the surface architecture of lymphocytes and their function. Polliack (*13–15*) believes that villous-covered lymphocytes represent B cells while cells with a smooth surface are T cells. Linthicum et al. (*12*) and Alexander and Wetzel (*1*), however, have shown that formation of villous projections is more a function of the method of cell preparation and has no correlation with cells being of bursal or thymic origin. In our study, villous-covered cells composed 70% of the lymphocytes in normal animals, with the remainder being smooth (18%) or possessing a few villi (12%).

LITERATURE CITED

1. Alexander, E. L. and B. Wetzel (1975). Human lymphocytes. Similarity of B and T cell surface morphology. Science 188:732–734.
2. Anderson, T. F. (1951). Techniques for preservation of 3-dimensional structure in preparing specimens for electron microscopy. Trans. N.Y. Acad. Sci. 13:130–134.
3. Chan, G., M. W. Rancourt, W. S. Ceglowski, and H. Friedman (1968). Leukemia virus suppression of antibody forming cells: Ultrastructure of infected spleen. Science 159:437–439.
4. deHarven, E., N. Lampen, T. Sato, and C. Friend (1973). Scanning electron microscopy of cells infected with a murine leukemia virus. Virology 51:240–243.
5. Friedman, H. and W. S. Ceglowski (1971). Nature and mechanism of tumor virus induced immunosuppression. Prog. Virol. 1:815–825.
6. Friedman, H. and J. R. Kately (1975). Lymphocyte surface receptors and leukemia virus-induced immunosuppression. Am. J. Clin. Pathol. 63:735–747.
7. Friend, C. (1957). Cell free transmission in adult Swiss mice of a disease having the character of a leukemia J. Exp. Med. 105:307–318.
8. Kately, J. R., J. Holderbach, and H. Friedman (1974). Leukemia virus-induced alteration of lymphocyte Ig surface receptors and the "capping" response of mouse spleen and lymph node cells. J. Nat. Cancer Inst. 53:1135–1140.
9. Koo, G. C., W. S. Ceglowski, and H. Friedman (1971). Immunosuppression by leukemia viruses. I. Ultrastructural studies of antibody forming spleen cells of mice infected with Friend leukemia virus. J. Immunol. 106:799–807.

10. Koo, G. C., W. S. Ceglowski, M. Higgins, and H. Friedman (1971). Immunosuppression by leukemia viruses. VI. Ultrastructure of individual antibody-forming cells in the spleens of friend leukemia virus infected mice. J. Immunol. 106:815–830.

11. Lin, P. S., A. G. Cooper, and H. H. Wortis (1973). Scanning electron microscopy of human T-cell and B-cell rose Hes. N. Engl. J. Med. 289:548–551.

12. Linthicum, S. S., S. Sell, R. M. Wagner, and P. Trefts (1974). Scanning immunoelectron microscopy of mouse B and T lymphocytes. Nature 253:173–175.

13. Polliack, A., N. Lampen, B. D. Clarkson, E. deHarven, A. Bentwich, F. P. Siegal, and H. G. Kunkel (1973). Identification of human B and T lymphocytes by scanning electron microscopy. J. Exp. Med. 138:607–624.

14. Polliack, A., S. M. Fu, S. D. Douglas, Z. Bentwich, N. Lampen, and E. deHarven (1974). Scanning electron microscopy of human lymphocyte-sheep erythrocyte rosettes. J. Exp. Med. 140:146–158.

15. Polliack, A., U. Hammerling, N. Lampen, and E. deHarven (1975). Surface morphology of murine B and T lymphocytes: A comparative study by scanning electron microscopy. Eur. J. Immunol. 5:32–39.

16. Rauscher, F. J. (1962). A virus induced disease of mice characterized by erthrocytopoiesis and lymphoid leukemia. J. Nat. Cancer Inst. 29:515–532.

17. Rich, M. A. and R. Siegler (1967). Virus leukemia in the mouse Ann. Rev. Microbiol. 21:529–572.

CHAPTER 15

Immunologic Control of Tumor Development in the Chicken

T. J. Linna, C. Hu,
K. M. Lam, and K. D. Thompson

I. INTRODUCTION

Much circumstantial evidence (*3, 4, 44*) favors the concept of a host-protective function for cell-mediated immunity in malignancy, although the evidence is by no means conclusive (*36, 37*). The role of the antibody-forming system in tumor development is even more controversial. In previous years much emphasis was given to the in vitro tumor-protective effect of tumor-bearer serum, and this effect was assumed to be due to "blocking" antibodies or antigen-antibody complexes (*12, 13*). While it seems that tumor-enhancing antibodies can be obtained using certain experimental protocols (*16, 17*), it seems that the "blocking" effect of tumor-bearer serum is mediated by tumor antigen, and when it is mediated by antigen-antibody complexes, they are in antigen excess (*1, 2*). These findings have radically changed the perspective on effects of the antibody-forming system on tumor development. Clinical (*19*) and experimental data (*14, 54*) now indicate that the antibody-forming system also has a host-protective function.

The chicken offers certain advantages in studies of influences of the immunologic system on tumor development because of the

These investigations were supported by the United States Public Health Service, National Institutes of Health grant CA 13347 from the National Cancer Institute, and by a National Institutes of Health General Research Support Grant to Temple University.

241

unique and fairly clear-cut delineation of immunologic responsiveness between cell-mediated, thymus-dependent immunity, and antibody-forming capacity, dependent on the bursa of Fabricius, a hindgut lymphoid organ unique for birds (7). Thus, thymectomy studies can be largely expected to elucidate the influence of cell-mediated immunity, and bursectomy studies the influence of antibody-forming system on tumor development. Treatment with immune serum on tumor-bearing and normal immunodeficient animals can be further expected to elucidate the influences of the antibody-forming system on tumor development. Studies in tumor systems of different genesis are necessary, if one wishes to claim that the phenomena are of general relevance in tumor immunology.

We report here results of studies with three avian tumor systems with regard to effects of the immunologic system on tumor development. Two of them are virus-induced, and will be dealt with in some detail. Since the third tumor system—a chemical carcinogen-induced transplantable tumor line—falls outside the main scope of this book, emphasizing tumor viruses, it will be dealt with only briefly.

The first avian tumor system studied by us in the context of immunologic control is the tumor caused by avian reticuloendotheliosis (RE) virus, strain T. This virus causes systemic (43, 52) and local (24) tumors. The tumor cells, first thought to be of lymphoid origin (43), have been shown to belong to the reticuloendothelial cell line (51). The RE virus is outside the avian leukosis-sarcoma complex, and is immunlogically and biochemically different from the avian tumor virus group (27, 34, 49). Data are presented below on the effects of thymectomy, bursectomy, and thymobursectomy on tumor development. We also present data on the efficacy of immune serum in the therapy of RE tumors. XC cells, a Rous sarcoma cell line carried in vitro for more than a decade in different laboratories, were originally derived from the tumor of a rat infected with the Prague strain of Rous sarcoma virus (45, 46). XC cells are known to contain the Rous Sarcoma genome, but they do not secrete the virus (47, 51). Administration of XC cells to chicken results in the appearance of sarcomatous tumors (20, 47). We present data on growth and incidence of XC cell-induced tumors, and on animal mortality from such tumors, in thymectomized, bursectomized, and control groups of birds.

Finally, some data are presented on the development of a benzo(a)pyrene-induced transplantable fibrosarcoma in thymectomized, bursectomized, and normal recipients. The data derived from these three widely different tumor models indicate clearly that both cell-mediated immunity and the antibody-forming system participate in the immune defense from malignancy.

II. EXPERIMENTAL DATA

Hy-Line WC chickens were used in all these studies. The surgical thymectomies and bursectomies were done on the day of hatching using the standard technique (35). Surgical bursectomy, even when performed on the day of hatching, does not regularly result in agammaglobulinemia and lack of antibody-forming capacity. Administration of high doses of cyclophosphamide to chickens in the newly hatched period has been demonstrated to result in agammaglobulinemia and lack of antibody-forming capacity at high frequency (21, 25), with concomitant destruction of the bursa of Fabricius and no permanent effect on cell-mediated immunity (25). Cyclophosphamide bursectomies were accomplished in this study by the intraperitoneal (i.p.) administration of 4 mg of cyclophosphamide daily during the first 3 days of life.

The RE virus, strain T, lethality was determined in normal chickens, which were inoculated intraperitoneally or into the wing web with varying doses of RE virus when 3 days old. The thymectomized animals and their controls received 5 LD_{50}s of RE virus into the wing web when 3 days old. The same schedule was used in the surgical bursectomy study. The cyclophosphamide-bursectomized animals were given 5 LD_{50}s of RE virus into the wing web at 1 month of age, i.e., when the immunodeficiency was specific for antibody-producing capacity (21, 25). The normal animals in the immune serum therapy experiments and their controls were given one LD_{50} into the wing web when 3 days old, and the cyclophosphamide-bursectomized animals in the serum study 1 LD_{50} into the wing web when 1 month old. In the thymobursectomy study, two doses of RE virus were used. Three-day-old animals were given 0.5 or 0.1 LD_{50} intraperitoneally.

Five million live (0.1% trypan blue-excluding) XC cells were administered into the wing web of thymectomized, bursectomized, or control recipients.

The transplantable tumor used in this study was raised in a thymectomized chicken using benzo(a)pyrene in trioactanoin and has a "take" frequency of about 100% when the major histocompatibility barrier is not crossed, and which is much lower across a major histocompatibility barrier.

Prospective immune serum donors were given 0.1 LD_{50} of RE virus into the wing web when 3 days old, challenged with 5 LD_{50}s of RE virus when 4 weeks old, and bled by cardiac puncture 6 weeks later. Serum was obtained in the usual manner, and decomplemented by heating at 56°C for 30 min. The portion of serum used for absorption of antiviral antibodies was absorbed with RE virus obtained from supernatants of virus-infected chick embryo fibroblast cultures.

Nonabsorbed antiserum was used to treat normal and cyclophosphamide-bursectomized chickens, which had received 1 LD_{50} of RE virus into the wing web 6 days earlier. At the time of the first injection, about 60% of the animals had measurable wing web tumors. A few days later, virtually all serum recipients were tumor bearing.

A. RE Virus Studies

1. Thymectomy Study   Development of progressively growing tumors, leading to death of the animals, occurred much more frequently in animals that were thymectomized in the newly hatched period and given RE virus into the wing web, than in the sham-operated animals, infected in the same way with RE virus (Table 1).

2. Bursectomy Studies   Both surgical bursectomy on the day of hatching, and chemical bursectomy, using high doses of cyclophosphamide in the newly hatched period (*21, 25*), led much more frequently to development of progressively growing, ultimately fatal tumors in the bursectomized birds, infected with RE virus into the wing web, than in the nonbursectomized, tumor virus-infected controls (Tables 2 and 3). More extensive information on the thymectomy studies and bursectomy studies can be found elsewhere (*24*).

Table 1. RE tumor development in thymectomized and sham-thymectomized chickens

Treatment	Regression of local tumors	Survivors
Thymectomy	13% (3/24)	8% (2/24)
	$p < 0.01$	$p < 0.002$
Sham-thymectomy	59% (13/22)	55% (12/22)

Table 2. RE tumor development in surgically bursectomized and normal chickens

Treatment	Regression of local tumors	Survivors
Surgical bursectomy	38% (8/21)	10% (2/21)
	$p < 0.05$	$p < 0.002$
Normal	76% (16/21)	62% (13/21)

Table 3. RE tumor development in cyclophosphamide bursectomized and normal chickens

Treatment	Regression of local tumors	Survivors
Cyclophosphamide bursectomy	50% (8/16)	12% (2/16)
	$p < 0.05$	$p < 0.002$
Normal	98% (16/18)	78% (15/18)

3. Thymo-bursectomy Studies   Tumor mortality was significantly higher in the groups that were surgically thymectomized and bursectomized on the day of hatching, and infected with RE virus intraperitoneally when 3 days old, than in the sham-operated, tumor virus-infected controls. When 0.1 LD_{50} of virus was used as the infecting dose, 64% (14/22) of the Tx-Bx chickens died of RE tumors and 32% (7/22) of the control birds died with tumors, $p < 0.05$. When 0.5 LD_{50} of virus was used as the infecting dose, 73% (16/22) of the treated chickens died with tumors, while only 32% (7/22) of the controls died with tumors, $p < 0.01$ (Table 4). Tumor mortality data in the control groups indicate that these experiments may have been very similar.

4. Immune Serum Therapy Studies   An intensive course of treatment of tumor-bearing normal animals with immune serum resulted in permanent regression of local tumors, and survival of the tumor virus-infected animals, significantly more frequently than in the normal serum-treated or nontreated controls. Actually, virtu-

Table 4. RE tumor mortality in surgically thymobursectomized chickens

Experiment	Controls	Tx–Bx	p
1	32% (7/22)	64% (14/22)	< 0.05
2	32% (7/22)	73% (16/22)	< 0.01

Table 5. Effect of normal and immune sera on the development of RE tumors in normal chickens

Treatment	Frequency of regression of local tumors	p	Frequency of survival	p
None	38% (6/16)		25% (4/16)	
Normal serum	19% (3/16)		19% (3/16)	
Immune serum	94% (15/16)	$< 0.01^a < 0.002^b$	94% (15/16)	$< 0.002^{a,b}$

[a]Comparison with no treatment.
[b]Comparison with normal serum treatment.

ally all immune serum-treated animals were able to regress their tumors and survive indefinitely, while virtually all normal serum-treated or nontreated animals died with progressively growing tumors (Table 5). To exclude the host-protective influence of the recipient's own antibody-forming system, similar studies were done in cyclophosphamide-bursectomized, tumor-bearing recipients. Again, treatment with immune serum resulted in permanent tumor regression and survival of virtually all treated animals, while virtually all nontreated and normal serum-treated animals died from progressively growing tumors. The differences were, again, statistically significant (Table 6).

Since the RE tumors are caused by an RNA tumor virus, the tumor cells produce RE virus, and the therapeutic effect of the immune serum could, at least partly, be due to antiviral antibodies. To study the influence of antiviral antibodies in tumor therapy in this system, the immune serum was extensively absorbed with RE virus. This treatment did not decrease the efficacy of immune serum in tumor therapy, demonstrating that the antiviral antibodies do not significantly contribute to tumor regression or animal survival in this experimental model (Table 7).

B.   XC Cell-induced Tumors

1. Thymectomy Study   Surgical thymectomy on the day of hatching resulted in significantly increased tumor frequency ($p <$ 0.02) (Table 8). Tumor mortality was also significantly higher in thymectomized ($p = 0.02$) than control birds (Figure 1). The XC cell-induced tumors grew at a much faster rate in thymectomized than in control animals, especially towards the end of the study (Figure 2).

2. Bursectomy Study   Surgical bursectomy on the day of hatching did not significantly influence tumor frequency or mortality; but in these animals, the tumors grew at a significantly faster rate than in controls, as documented by significantly larger tumor sizes ($p < 0.01$) in bursectomized animals towards the end of the experiments by analysis of variance (Table 8 and Figures 1 and 2).

C.   Benzo(*a*)pyrene-induced Transplantable Tumors

1. Thymectomy and Bursectomy Studies   Thymectomy on the day of hatching did not significantly affect tumor frequency or growth rate in this study. On the other hand, when animals were surgically bursectomized on the day of hatching and inoculated with

Table 6. Effect of normal and immune sera on the development of the RE tumors in cyclophosphamide-bursectomized chickens

Treatment	Frequency of regression of local tumors	p	Frequency of survival	p
None	50% (8/16)		12% (2/16)	
Normal serum	53% (10/19)		37% (7/19)	
Immune serum	90% (18/20)	< 0.05[a]	90% (18/20)	< 0.01[a]

[a]Comparison with no treatment or normal serum treatment.

Table 7. Effect of nonabsorbed and absorbed immune sera on the development of RE tumors

Treatment	Frequency of regression of local tumors	p	Frequency of survival	p
None	23% (3/13)		15% (2/13)	
Nonabsorbed immune serum	65% (11/17)	N.S.[a]	59% (10/17)	< 0.05[a]
Absorbed immune serum	80% (12/15)	< 0.02[a]	73% (11/15)	< 0.01[a]

[a]Comparison with no treatment.

Table 8. Incidence of tumors in thymectomized, bursectomized, and control chickens inoculated with XC cells

Treatment	No. of chickens	No. of chickens with tumors	Percentage
Thymectomy	26	25	96[a]
Bursectomy	25	16	64
Control	22	14	63

[a]Significantly higher ($p < 0.02$) when compared with controls (Fisher's exact test).

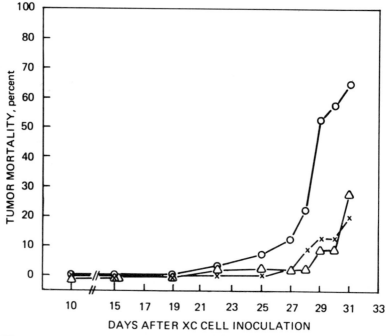

Figure 1. Cumulative mortality of thymectomized, $\times - \times$, bursectomized, $\bigcirc - \bigcirc$, and control, $\triangle - \triangle$, chickens inoculated with XC cells.

tumor cells on the third day, there was no clear difference in tumor frequency between bursectomized and control animals. However, the bursectomized animals had significantly ($p < 0.01$) larger tumors than controls toward the end of the observation period, as evaluated by Student's t-test. Upon closer examination with multivariate profile analysis, tumor growth rate was found to be significantly ($p < 0.005$) faster in bursectomized than in control birds (Figure 3).

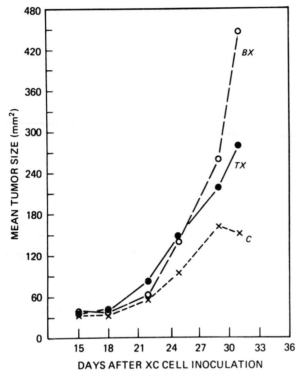

Figure 2. Mean tumor sizes of thymectomized, (Tx), bursectomized, (Bx), and control, (c), chickens inoculated with XC cells.

III.   DISCUSSION

The unique and fairly well-defined delineation of immunologic responsiveness in the chicken into thymus-dependent, cell-mediated immunity on one hand, and bursa-dependent, humoral immunity on the other (7) makes this species especially attractive for studies of the separate influences of cell-mediated immunity and of the antibody-forming system on tumor development in vivo. While the in vitro methods have provided much useful insight into the mechanisms by which lymphoid cells and/or antibodies can effect tumor target cells (6, 26, 33), the acid test of the relevance of such mechanisms is the demonstration of these mechanisms in vivo. We have studied these influences in the chicken model, and report here results from such studies in three tumors of widely different genesis, namely: (1) avian reticuloendotheliosis, caused by an RNA tumor virus outside

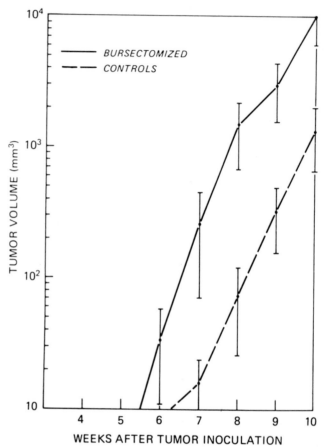

Figure 3. Mean BP-1 tumor volume in bursectomized and control chickens.

the avian leukosis-sarcoma complex; (2) tumors induced by XC cells, a Rous sarcoma-derived tumor line; and (3) a benzo(*a*)pyrene-induced transplantable fibrosarcoma. Thymectomy has been shown to result in a decreased capacity of the host to defend itself against the malignancy for both virus-induced tumors, while surgical thymectomy alone in the newly hatched period has not been found to influence significantly the development of the transplantable tumor line (*22*). The question of whether more stringent experimental ablation of the thymus and the T-cell system would influence the development of this chemical carcinogen-induced tumor line falls outside the scope of this chapter. Suffice it to state that the data obtained with the virus-induced tumors support the concept of a host-protective "surveillance" function for cell-mediated immunity.

The data obtained for the influence of the bursa of Fabricius and the antibody-forming system on tumor development clearly demonstrate that the bursa-dependent, antibody-forming system has a host-protective influence on all three tumors studied—a "surveillance" function. The data are most extensive for the RE virus-induced tumors, and demonstrate that surgical or chemical bursectomy with impairment of the antibody-forming capacity increases tumor frequency, mortality, and progression. Immune serum can cause regression and cure of RE virus-induced tumors, apparently by action of antibodies, since this immune serum has no effect on development of tumors caused by a laboratory strain of Marek's disease, and the effect can be reproduced by administration of the λ-globulin fraction obtained from immune serum, but not from normal serum. The antibodies are probably directed against transplantation-type antigens on tumor cells, since extensive absorption of antiviral antibodies does not decrease the efficacy of immune serum in tumor cure.

The studies of RE tumor development in animals that had undergone combined bursectomy and thymectomy on the day of hatching are of interest, since they illustrate the effect of deficiency of both cell-mediated and humoral immunity on tumor development. These studies demonstrate that the combined immunodeficiency increases tumor mortality. It is not possible to compare the results from these studies with those of thymectomy or bursectomy alone, since they were not done parallel with the thymobursectomy studies, and the experimental conditions do not permit comparisons between studies done at different times. The fact remains that tumor mortality in thymobursectomized animals was significantly higher than in sham-operated controls, indicating a host-protective influence of the immune system as a whole. The data seem to argue against the immunostimulation hypothesis (36, 37) since an absence of immunologic reactivity would also mean an absence of the tumor-stimulating effect of immunity. However, this interpretation is by no means certain, since the absence of antiviral antibodies may have increased the ability of the tumor virus to reach target cells. Also, surgical thymobursectomy may not have crippled immunity completely in the newly hatched period without adjunct treatment. Some degree of immunologic reactivity may remain, which could even stimulate

254 Linna et al.

tumor development. Thus, this study does not provide adequate information on the biologic relevance of the immunostimulation concept.

The RE virus is an unusual tumor virus. It is outside the avian leukosis-sarcoma group, based on immunologic (51) and biochemical (27) studies. Although the disease studied by us is clearly a malignancy, as judged by its morphology and ability to grow invasively (48, 51), formation of local tumors after local RE virus administration, and the presence of a virus-induced cell line causing tumors in vivo (11), some members of the reticuloendotheliosis virus group cause lytic lesions without a tumor component (50). Therefore, we extended our studies of the influence of cell-mediated and of humoral immunity on tumor development into another avian tumor virus system.

We turned our attention to Rous sarcoma, a classic virus group in the avian tumor virus complex. Since both Bryan strain (28) and Carr-Zilber strain (40) have been studied with regard to effect of bursectomy and agammaglobulinemia on tumor development with essentially negative results, we took another approach. XC cells were used to obtain tumor development. XC cells, widely used in vitro studies in virology, are derived from the tumor of a rat inoculated with the Prague strain of Rous sarcoma virus (RSV). XC cells contain the RSV genome but do not contain or secrete virus. RSV can be recovered from XC cells after cocultivation with chick embryo fibroblasts. Inoculation with XC cells, or with the supernatant of the mixture of XC cells and chick embryo fibroblasts, can induce sarcomatous tumors in chickens. In both cases, infectious RSV is formed and released (45, 46). XC cells were administered into wing webs of chickens that were surgically bursectomized or thymectomized in the newly hatched period, or were untreated. Thymectomy resulted in significantly higher tumor frequency and mortality, and also in significantly larger tumors (Table 8, Figures 1 and 2). Surgical bursectomy had a significant influence on tumor size in this study, but not on the other parameters studied (Figure 2). Thus, influence of immunity on tumor development can be demonstrated also in this virus-induced tumor system. In this case, as in the case of the benzo(a)pyrene-induced transplantable tumor, bursectomy influenced tumor size rather than "take" or frequency (Figure 3). Since data on a more complete ablation of the bursa-dependent system are not available at present, we do not know if such treatment would also influence parameters other than tumor growth rate.

Thus, we have demonstrated that not only cell-mediated immunity, but also the antibody-forming system plays a host-protective role in two different virus-induced malignancies. A similar function for the antibody-forming system was also shown in a third, chemical carcinogen-induced, transplantable tumor system. With similar data in three avian malignancies of widely different genesis, it seems feasible to propose that the bursa-dependent, antibody-forming system may play a host-protective role in malignancy in general. Data presented here and elsewhere (23, 24, 52) certainly support such a concept. In the case of Marek's disease, a DNA virus-induced malignancy, published data indicate that thymectomy does not greatly influence the development of this tumor (10). However, since most tumor cells (at least in some laboratory strains of Marek's disease) seem to be T cells (15, 42), thymectomy experiments are difficult to interpret clearly. That is, the manipulation can affect both the virus target cell population and the population involved in cell-mediated immunologic defenses, and these influences could counteract each other. Data on the effects of bursectomy on development of Marek's disease are inconclusive and controversial (18, 30, 32, 42). Although some degree of host protection by passively transferred antibodies has been reported (5), the role played by humoral immunity in host resistance in Marek's disease remains to be determined. The efficacy of turkey herpesvirus vaccine in protection from Marek's disease has been amply documented (31, 38, 53). The role of immunity in this protection is unclear (8, 39), although the antibody-forming system may contribute to this protection (39).

In recent years, much emphasis has been placed on tumor enhancement by serum components, presumed to be antibodies or antigen-antibody complexes in birds (5) and mammals, including man (12, 13). It is becoming increasingly clear that this enhancement is due to circulating tumor antigen, and when it is due to antigen-antibody complexes, they are in antigen excess (1, 2). Evidence for a host-protective function of the antibody-forming system in certain malignancies is well documented in the older literature (31, 53) as well as in recent data (14).

Thus, we have found evidence for a host-protective "surveillance" function by cell-mediated immunity and by the antibody-forming system in vivo for widely different tumors. Support for this concept can also be found in the literature. These immunologic mechanisms can work separately or in concert, in addition to other host-protective mechanisms, e.g., the macrophage system (9, 38). The biologic significance of these mechanisms in malignancy in general is presently uncertain and probably varies with different tumors. However, the fact that immunologic mechanisms can be shown to have a host-protective function, at least in certain malignancies, gives hope that the aid of immunity can be used in tumor prevention and cure.

ACKNOWLEDGMENTS

We thank Miss Annsofi Holst and Mr. Robert Kalwinski for technical assistance.

LITERATURE CITED

1. Alexander, P. (1974). Escape from immune destruction by the host through shedding of surface antigens: Is this a characteristic shared by malignant and embryonic cells? Cancer Res. 34:2077–2082.
2. Baldwin, R. W., J. G. Bowen, and M. R. Price (1973). Detection of circulating hepatoma D23 antigen and immune complexes in tumor bearing serum. Br. J. Cancer 28:16–24.
3. Burnet, F. M. (1970). The concept of immunological surveillance. Prog. Exp. Tumor Res. 13:1–27.
4. Burnet, F. M. (1970). Immunological Surveillance. Pergamon Press, Oxford.
5. Calnek, B. W. (1972). Effects of passive antibody on early pathogenesis of Marek's disease. Infect. Immunity 6:193–198.
6. Cerottini, J. C. and K. T. Brunner (1974). Cell-mediated cytotoxicity, allograft refection and immunity. Adv. Immunol. 18:67–132.
7. Cooper, M. D., R. D. A. Peterson, M. A. South, and R. A. Good (1966). The function of the thymus system and bursa system in the chicken. J. Exp. Med. 123:75–102.
8. Else, R. W. (1974). Vaccinal immunity to Marek's disease in bursectomized chickens. Vet. Rec. 95:182–187.
9. Evans, R., H. Cox, and P. Alexander (1973). Immunologically specific activation of macrophages armed with the specific macrophage arming factor (SMAF). Proc. Soc. Exp. Biol. Med. 143:256–259.
10. Foster, A. G., and T. Moll (1968). Effect of immunosuppression on clinical and pathologic manifestations of Marek's disease in chickens. Am. J. Vet. Res. 29:1831–1835.

11. Franklin, R. B., R. L. Maldonado, and H. R. Bose (1974). Isolation and characterization of reticuloendotheliosis virus in transformed bone marrow cells. Intervirology 3:342–352.

12. Hellstrom, K. E. and I. Hellstrom (1970). Immunological enhancement as studied by cell culture techniques. Ann. Rev. Microbiol. 24:373–398.

13. Hellstrom, K. E. and I. Hellstrom (1974). Lymphocyte-mediated cytotoxicity and blocking serum activity to tumor antigens. Adv. Immunol. 18:209–277.

14. Hersey, P. (1973). The protective effect of antisera against leukemia in vivo—A reappraisal. Br. J. Cancer 28:Suppl. I, 11–18.

15. Hudson, L. and L. N. Payne (1973). An analysis of the T and B cells in Marke's disease lymphomas of the chicken. Nature (New Biol.) 241:52–53.

16. Kaliss, N. (1958). Immunological enhancement of tumor homografts in mice. Cancer Res. 18:992–1003.

17. Kaliss, N. and F. W. Fitch (1971). Immunological enhancement. In: Progress in Immunology, B. Amos, Ed., Vol. I. Academic Press, New York.

18. Kenyon, A. J., M. Sevoian, M. Horwitz, N. J. Jones, and C. F. Helmboldt (1969). Lymphoproliferative disease of fowl-immunological factors associated with passage of a lymphoblastic leukemia (JM-V). Avain Dis. 13:585–595.

19. Kersey, J. H., B. D. Spector, and R. A. Good (1973). Primary immunodeficiency disease and cancer: The immunodeficiency-cancer registry. Int. J. Cancer 12:333–347.

20. Lam, K. M. and T. J. Linna (1975). Effect of thymectomy and bursectomy on XC cell-induced tumors in chickens. Fed. Proc. 34:852.

21. Lerman, S. P. and W. P. Weidanz (1970). The effect of cyclophosphamide on the ontogeny of the humoral immune response in chickens. J. Immunol. 105:614–619.

22. Linna, T. J. (1975). Increased growth rate of a Benzo(a)pyrene-induced transplantable tumor in bursectomized chickens. Fed. Proc. 34:963.

23. Linna, T. J. and C. Hu (1975). Roles of cellular and humoral immunity in malignancy. In: O. F. Nygaard, H. I. Adler, and W. K. Sinclair, (eds.), Radiation Research. p. 909–916. Academic Press, New York.

24. Linna, T. J., C. Hu, and K. D. Thompson (1974). Development of systemic and local tumors induced by avian reticuloendotheliosis virus after thymectomy or bursectomy. J. Nat. Cancer Inst. 53:847–854.

25. Linna, T. J., D. Frommel, and R. A. Good (1972). Effects of early cyclophosphamide treatment on the development of lymphoid organs and immunological functions in the chicken. Int. Arch. Allergy 42:20–39.

26. MacLennan, I. C. M. (1972). Antibody in the induction and inhibition of lymphocyte cytotoxicity. Transplant. Rev. 13:67–90.

27. Maldonado, R. L. and H. R. Bose (1973). Relationship of reticuloendotheliosis virus to the avian tumor viruses: Nucleic acid and polypeptide composition. J. Virol. 11:741–747.
28. McArthur, W. P., E. A. Carwell and G. J. Thorbecke (1972). Growth of Rous sarcomas in bursectomized chickens. J. Nat. Cancer Inst. 49:907–909.
29. Morrison, D. F. (1967). Multivariate Statistical Methods. McGraw-Hill, New York.
30. Morris, J. R., F. N. Jerome, and B. S. Reinhart (1969). Surgical bursectomy and the incidence of Marek's disease (MD) in domestic chickens. Poultry Sci. 48:1513–1515.
31. Okazaki, W., H. G. Purchase, and B. R. Burmester (1970). Protection against Marek's disease by vaccination with a herpes virus of turkeys. Avian Dis. 14:413–429.
32. Payne, L. N. and M. J. Rennie (1970). Effect of bursectomy on Marek's disease. J. Nat. Cancer Inst. 45:387–397.
33. Perlman, P., H. Perlman, and H. Wigzell (1973). Lymphocyte mediated cytotoxicity in vitro. Induction and inhibition by humoral antibody and nature of effector cells. Transplant. Rev. 13:91–114.
34. Peterson, D. A., K. L. Baxter-Gabbard, and A. S. Levine (1972). Avian reticuloendotheliosis virus (strain T.) V. DNA polymerase. Virology 47:251–254.
35. Peterson, R. D. A., B. R. Burmester, T. N. Frederickson, H. G. Purchase, and R. A. Good (1964). Effect of bursectomy and thymectomy on the development of visceral lymphomatosis in the chicken. J. Nat. Cancer Inst. 32:1343–1354.
36. Prehn, R. T. (1971). Perspectives on oncogenesis: Does immunity stimulate or inhibit neoplasia? J. Reticuloendothel. Soc. 10:1–16.
37. Prehn, R. T. 1972. The immune reaction as a stimulator of tumor growth. Science 176:170–171.
38. Purchase, H. G., W. Okazaki, and B. R. Burmester (1972). Long-term field trials with the herpesvirus of turkeys vaccine against Marek's disease. Avian Dis. 16:57–71.
39. Purchase, H. G. and J. M. Sharma (1974). Amelioration of Marek's disease and absence of vaccine protection in immunologically deficient chickens. Nature 248:419–421.
40. Radzichovskaja, R. (1967). Effect of bursectomy on the Rous virus tumor induction in chickens. Nature 213:1259–1260.
41. Reed, L. J. and H. Muench (1938). A simple method of estimating fifty percent end points. Am. J. Hyg. 27:493–497.
42. Rouse, B. T., R. J. H. Wells, and N. L. Warner (1973). Proportion of T and B lymphocytes in lesions of Marek's disease: Theoretical implications for pathogenesis. J. Immunol. 110:534–539.
43. Sevoian, M., R. N. Larose, and D. M. Chamberlain (1964). Avian lymphomatosis. VI. A virus of unusual potency and pathogenicity. Avian Dis. 8:336–347.
44. Smith, R. T. and M. Landy, Eds. (1970). Immune Surveillance. Academic Press, New York.

45. Svoboda, J. (1960). Presence of chicken tumour virus in the sarcoma of the adult rat inoculated after birth with Rous sarcoma tissue. Nature 186:980–981.
46. Svoboda, J. (1961). The tumorigenic action of Rous sarcoma in rats and the permanent production of Rous virus by the induced rat sarcoma XC. Folia Biol. (Praha) 7:46–70.
47. Svoboda, J., P. Chyle, D. Simkovic, and I. Hilgert (1963). Demonstration of the absence of infectious Rous virus in rat tumor XC whose structurally intact cells produce Rous sarcoma virus when transferred to chickens. Folia Biol. (Praha) 9:77–81.
48. Taylor, H. W. and L. D. Olson (1973). Chronologic study of the T-virus in chicks. I. Development of lesions. Avian Dis. 17:782–794.
49. Temin, H. M. (1974). On the origin of the genes for neoplasia. Cancer Res. 34:2835–2841.
50. Temin, H. M. and V. K. Kassner (1974). Replication of reticuloendotheliosis viruses in culture: Acute infection. J. Virol. 13:291–297.
51. Theilen, G. H., R. F. Zeigel, and M. J. Twiehaus (1966). Biological studies with RE virus (Strain T) that induces reticuloendotheliosis in turkeys, chickens and Japanese quail. J. Nat. Cancer Inst. 37:731–742.
52. Thompson, K. D. and T. J. Linna (1973). Bursa-dependent "surveillance" of a virus-induced tumor in the chicken. Nature New Biol. 245:10–12.
53. Witter, R. L., K. Nazerian, H. G. Purchase, and G. H. Burgoyne (1970). Isolation from turkeys of a cell-associated herpesvirus antigenically related to Marek's disease virus. Am. J. Vet. Res. 31:525–538.
54. Woodruff, M., N. Dunbar, and A. Ghaffar (1973). The growth of tumors in T-cell derived mice and their response to treatment with *Corynebacterium parvum*. Proc. Roy. Soc. London B 184:97–102.

CHAPTER 16

Immunotherapy of Experimental Cancer with BCG

H. J. Rapp

Immunotherapy of human cancer with *Mycobacterium bovis,* strain BCG, is now being investigated in several clinical centers (*1*). Studies with a guinea pig hepatoma model have been helpful in interpreting the results of some clinical investigations and may be useful as a guide in the design of new clinical trials (*3*). Many patients with multiple cutaneous metastases of recurrent malignant melanoma have been treated by the intralesional injection of BCG. In more than half of these patients, injected lesions have regressed. Patients whose injected lesions did not regress were usually in a far advanced stage of the disease and had evidence of depressed immunity. In about 15% of patients, uninjected lesions as well as injected lesions regressed. This observation is consistent with the finding in the guinea pig hepatoma studies that a single injection of BCG into a tumor growing in the skin not only causes the injected tumor to regress but also eradicates lymph node metastases. Permanent cures in the guinea pig model are obtained if BCG is given at a time when there are microscopic metastases. Treatment at a time when there are palpable metastases, however, is at best palliative. This finding is consistent with the fact that treatment of recurrent malignant human melanoma with intralesional BCG is palliative but has rarely resulted in cures or even prolongation of life. According to the guinea pig model, there would be hope of permanent cures of human malignant melanoma if the primary early disease rather than the recurrent disease were treated by the intralesional injection of BCG before surgery or other forms of therapy. A clinical study to test this prediction is now in progress at the National Cancer Institute.

The guinea pig immunotherapy model was an outgrowth of basic studies of tumor immunology with the objective of demonstrating tumor-specific immunity by the delayed cutaneous hypersensitivity (DCH) reaction. Hepatomas were induced in inbred, strain-2, guinea pigs by administration of diethylnitrosamine in drinking water. Several transplantable tumor lines were developed and maintained in the ascites form by adapting the neoplasms to grow in the peritoneal cavity. Inoculation of viable cells from any of these lines intraperitoneally or intramuscularly caused lethal, metastatic malignant disease. There were, however, major differences among these lines in the growth characteristics of tumors resulting from the intradermal inoculation of tumor cells. Line 1, for example, produced skin tumors that grew for a few days and then regressed. After the line 1 skin tumors regressed, the animals were found to be immune to systemic challenge with this tumor. Line 7, on the other hand, grew progressively in the skin but did not metastasize readily from this site. Animals could be immunized against line 7 by surgical excision of the skin tumor. Line 10 also grew progressively in the skin but metastasized readily to lymph nodes. This tumor has been used extensively as a model for studies on the immunotherapy of cancer. Initial attempts to demonstrate the development of tumor immunity against line 10 failed. Basic studies on the antigenicity of the different tumor lines led to the development of methods to immunize guinea pigs against line 10, and to eradicate established tumors as well as metastases.

In agreement with previous studies in mice, it was found that the guinea pig tumor lines each had individually specific transplantation antigens. With one particular pair of tumors, however, it was possible to cause rejection of one of the tumors in animals that were not immunized against that tumor. This rejection occurred in guinea pigs that had been immunized against a tumor antigenically unrelated to the first one, provided that the two tumors were mixed together and injected intradermally at the same site. The first tumor was not rejected when it was injected alone into animals immunized against the unrelated tumor. This observation suggested the possibility that the immunologic rejection of tumors in part may be due to reactions not requiring specific tumor immunity. This apparently nonspecific rejection of tumor growth was associated with the development of immunologically specific inflammation (delayed cutaneous hypersensitivity) against the tumor used for immunization. From this and other lines of evidence it was postulated that macrophages were important in this so-called "innocent bystander" effect. For relevance to the treatment of human cancer, however, it was necessary to find methods to eradicate established, palpable tumors and metastases rather than merely prevent the outgrowth of a few tumor cells in a challenge inoculum.

The hepatoma designated line 10 was used in these studies because within 7 days following intradermal injection of line 10 cells, there were invariably metastases to the draining lymph node. Conventional methods used in attempts to induce specific immunity against line 10 failed. Intradermal injection of a mixture consisting of line 10 cells and living BCG, however, rendered animals specifically resistant to challenge with this tumor. Previously, several methods had been used to induce inflammation at the sites of established line 10 tumors growing in the skin, but the tumors did not regress. When living BCG was injected directly into the growing tumor, however, the tumors in most treated animals became necrotic and eventually disappeared, and the animals remained tumor-free during periods of observation up to 3 years. Permanent cures were obtained even when treatment was started a time when there were metastatic cells in the draining lymph node.

Studies aimed at uncovering the mechanism of action of intralesionally administered BCG against established tumors have yielded little information beyond a superficial description of the accompanying events. Within 1 week after BCG is injected into the dermal tumor, there is a marked inflammatory reaction in and around the injection site which becomes necrotic and eventually heals. The healed site and the draining lymph node are free of tumor cells. The inflammatory response to BCG is, at least in part, mediated by small lymphocytes specifically sensitized against BCG antigens. When these lymphocytes encounter and react with these antigens, they release migration inhibition factor (MIF), a lymphokine that immobilizes macrophages. Since the BCG was injected into the tumor, the highest concentration of MIF will be present in the tumor and therefore macrophages will congregate at that site. It is likely that the immobilized macrophages are responsible for the necrosis associated with destruction of the tumor. One may speculate that the macrophages process tumor-specific antigen in a way that permits the host to acquire specific resistance to the tumor. Animals with specific resistance against line 10 possess small lymphocytes that can be used to transfer this resistance to unimmunized recipients. It is highly probable that these lymphocytes are responsible for the maintenance of long-term cures by eliminating or helping to eliminate tumor cells at metastatic sites.

Attempts to find in vitro measures of tumor immunity that correlate with long-term cure have failed. These in vitro measures include tumor antigen-mediated lymphocyte proliferation and tumor cell killing (2). While these and other reactivities can easily be demonstrated in animals after the intralesional injection of BCG, their presence or absence does not correlate with cure or lack of cure. The results of an experiment summarized in Table 1 show that even the development of tumor-specific delayed cutaneous hypersensitivity does not necessarily ensure that the animal will be cured. Although little is known about how intralesional BCG destroys established tumors and metastases, it is likely that this agent will be of importance in the control of human cancer.

Table 1. Lack of correlation between tumor-specific delayed cutaneous hypersensitivity and tumor immunity

Treatment of 7-day tumors with BCG, route of injection 12/31/74	Challenge with live tumor cells intradermally on day 28, mm induration on day 29	No. of animals that rejected tumor challenge	No. of animals with lymph node metastases
		No. tested 3/31/75	No. tested 3/31/75
Intratumor	7.2 ± 0.44	7/8	0/16
Intrafootpad (tumors in both groups excised on day 14)	6.4 ± 0.48	0/8	16/16

LITERATURE CITED

1. Bast, R. C., Jr., B. Zbar, T. Borsos, and H. J. Rapp (1974). BCG and Cancer. N. Engl. J. Med. 290:1413–1420; 1458–1469.
2. Littman, B. H., M. S. Meltzer, R. P. Cleveland, B. Zbar, and H. J. Rapp (1973). Tumor specific cell-mediated immunity in guinea pigs with tumors. J. Nat. Cancer Inst. 51:1627–1635.
3. Rapp, H. J. (1973). A guinea pig model for tumor immunology. A summary. Israel J. Med. Sci. 9:366–374.

Index